To My Precious Sister
Lucy,

# Enforcing Grace

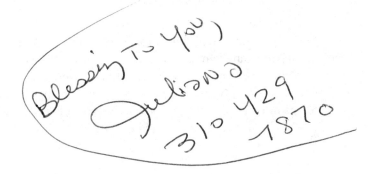

Blessing To You)
Juliana
310 429 1870

*"The kingdom of heaven suffereth violence and the violent take it by force."* (Matthew 11:12)

Rev. Juliana Taylor, Ph.D.

ISBN-13: 978-1-4507-5439-2

Manufactured in the United States of America

First Edition

*This book is dedicated to every soul seeking healing,*

*every heart seeking a deeper connection to God,*

*and every human spirit's right to divine health*

*on earth, here and now. Grace be with you.*

# ACKNOWLEDGMENTS

This testimony wouldn't have been possible without Pastor Henry Wright of Restoration Ministries, who had the courage and integrity to be led by the spirit and do the will of the Lord. I want to thank all of God's vessels who were in His service and were chosen to partake in my healing, including Sisters Rachel, Lynn, Donna and Nellie. These wonderful women stood with me, prayed for me, and rejoiced with me in my victories.

My special gratitude goes to my Sister in the Lord, Nellie, who imparted her faith, wisdom, and understanding of the deeper ways of the Lord. *"The effectual fervent prayers of a righteous servant availeth much."* (James 5:16)

She, as a consecrated vessel of God, was in agreement with one immutable fact: *"The entrance of His Word giveth light ..."* (Psalm 119:30)

# PREFACE

The message of this book is simple. You already have God's grace. There is no way to earn it, and it cannot be gotten through the works of religion. God's grace is sufficient! (2 Corinthians 12:9)

This all-encompassing grace is inclusive for the healing of all illnesses: spiritual, mental and emotional.

We, as the beloved children of the Great I Am, have a divine right to appropriate and enforce the grace of God through the action of retaliation faith. We take back what God has freely given us and become who we truly are ... the righteousness of God in Christ!

# CONTENTS

# INTRODUCTION

In her eleventh hour…

Rev. Dr. Juliana Taylor was resurrected from her deathbed after she was diagnosed with terminal lupus and environmental illness. She had become allergic to all foods and all chemicals, and spent years living in total isolation.

She was unable to wear clothing or sleep on normal bedding material.

She was sixty pounds, despondent and suicidal, when she was told she would never recover. Faced with these facts, even doctors from renowned worldwide clinics (immune system specialists) knew that they were powerless and that their treatments had been ineffective.

It was from this place of utter victimization and despair that Juliana had a Damascus experience with the Lord. The "Great Physician" arrived with a revelation on His purpose and intent for her life!

Alone in her living room, Juliana received the revelation on healing that would begin her new faith walk. She was told that she would learn to appropriate her miracle healing via her authority in Christ.

She soon discovered the type of faith that would expedite miracle healing was the faith of "divine retaliation."

We are invited on her journey as this empowering story unfolds and Rev. Juliana becomes the spiritual person that God intended her to be: the new creature in Christ, the eternal, immortal spirit complete in Him, with authority over her body, thoughts and emotions. *"If any man be in Christ, he is a new creature, old things are passed away, all things have become new." (Corinthians 6:17)*

Picking up the "Sword of the Spirit," she slays idol after idol, violently attacking her oppressions and deceptions. *"And take the helmet of salvation and the sword of the spirit, which is the word of God." (Ephesians 6:17)*

The miracles that we read about in this testimony are evoked by the primal and simple spiritual action of divine retaliation.

This testimony reveals how a sick and dying woman steps out of utter helplessness, abandonment and isolation and is healed in an absolute and extraordinary surrender to God, only to find out that her surrender is a baby step and insufficient to maintain her healing. She is unable to hold on to her God-given miracle! A battle unfolds.

This battle is called the battle between the flesh and the spirit. *"For the flesh lusteth against the spirit and the spirit against the flesh." (Galatians 5:17)* This is the battle we are all in on this earth, without exception! *"For we are the circumcision, which worship God in the spirit, and rejoice in Christ Jesus, and have no confidence in the flesh." (Philippians 3:3)*

We join Juliana as she takes back her proper identity in Christ. We become inspired as we are participants of a demonstration of spiritual regeneration that heals body, mind and soul. *"Not by the works of righteousness but according to His mercy He saved us, by the washing of regeneration, and the renewing of the Holy Ghost." (Titus 3:5)*

We begin to clearly perceive that no more do we as Christians need to hang around passively waiting and begging to be healed. The Lord Jesus Christ has conquered the law of sin and death. *"And having spoiled principalities and powers he made a show of them openly triumphing over them in it." (Colossians 2:15)*

This was a demonstration of total spiritual dominion! All power had been given unto Him in heaven and on earth!

On page 198, Dr. Taylor instructs, "The curse of the law has been broken. The law has no power over you! The Cross of Christ was not suffered in vain." *The old nature is faking its authority over you, she explains, and you can call its bluff!*

Your illnesses, pains and heartaches are the con job of the old nature itself. It simply does not belong to you! Your healing was provided for you at the Cross of Calvary. *"And you, hath he quickened together with him, having forgiven you all tres- passes." (Colossians 3:13)*

Dr. Taylor feels that the authority and power in Christ is available to all; it is here to be taken. That may be the only way to apprehend it! *"The Kingdom of heaven suffereth violence and the violent take it by force." (Matthew 11:12)*

We as "Retaliators in Christ" are separating ourselves from deceptions that would otherwise undermine our God-given inheritance and identity, our dominion that has already been fully and completely established for us on earth. *"But if ye are led of the spirit ye are not under the law." (Galatians 6:18)*

If you are reading this book and you are a person of faith, there is not one reason on this earth that you cannot be healed. Healing is available to you now — today. By His stripes ye were healed.

*A "retaliator" is simply an enforcer of the grace of God!*

Many have been healed just by reading these revelations and testimonies. Many have been healed by applying the miracle- working power of enforcing grace in their own lives.

Dr. Taylor now ministers in miracle-healing services world- wide; she has been commissioned to bring God's people out of the law of sin and death (sin consciousness, condemnation and guilt) into a prophetic end-time movement of freedom and authority in the spirit of life in Christ Jesus.

*Out of religion and into the fullness, depth and authenticity of life in the spirit. This includes divine health!*

She has noticed that the terms we use to enforce His grace are irrelevant to God. As long as we are "calling the bluff" of the con that is presenting evidence contrary to our divine health, authority and peace on this earth, we will have the victory. Whether you believe this "bluff" is of the carnal mind, ego, impostor, mortal mind, evil, generational principalities or devils, it really doesn't matter — as long as we do not allow how we see it or name it to stop us from taking right action.

It is only when we are seduced into agreeing with our "oppressor" and deceived into embracing our inner child, loving our ego, or fixing our inner self, that we will not be healed.

Dr. Taylor continues to stand and enforce His word in her personal life and ministry, and believes that living large and radically alive in the spirit of Christ and in His freedom and authority is a great worship unto the Lord.

> *"The law of the spirit of life in Christ Jesus hath set me free from the law of sin and death." (Romans 8:2)*

# Chapter 1

## Not One More Powerless Day

I had become a tormented and tortured creature, living in utter isolation in a small, bare, natural wood cabin in the Santa Barbara mountains.

I had no presentable clothing and no furniture, with the exception of a glass table that I slept on and an old wooden rocking chair upon which I sat.

When I looked in the mirror, I felt shame at my reflection. I did not recognize myself! Who was this creature peering back at me? This could not be me! How could this have happened?

I had once been an attractive woman, a model, a dancer and an actress. I had become a psychologist with the money earned from a successful acting career.

Whoever this impostor was, she was unidentifiable. I had no interest in her future. It was over. I had lost too many battles. There was no hope of regaining any strength. The war had been for my identity, and my identity had been overcome.

I would not give this impostor the last round. I would no longer submit to this master. There was no reason to! I had hit my personal bottom. I was as low as a human being could go and still be alive.

I hadn't always been this victimized!

Once I had been on higher ground. I had walked with God, the creator of Heaven and Earth. That loss was much more disturbing to me than my appearance, or even my lost health. I had lost my connection to God. That was the real issue! I couldn't hear my maker. The Spirit couldn't lead me. I was in darkness. I was dying in the wilderness.

I would not wither away and die a slow, tormented death. I would not wait around to be totally diminished. I decided to take action while I still had the ability to do so.

I looked directly into the impostor's eyes — eyes whose expression no longer belonged to me, eyes that were disconnected from my heart.

"I may be down," I heard myself say, "but I am not taking it anymore. I've had it. I refuse to live one more powerless day! Not one more powerless day!"

## You Will Not Kill Me!

As I heard my own defiant words, a rage rose up from within me. My voice deepened, and I spoke from a very primal place! "You will not kill me. You will not! I will kill you!"

She was still staring at me, her hair white, wild and brittle. Once my hair had been lovely, long, blond and full. I touched her mane. It was coarse and dry. The hand that touched her hair was foreign to me. Lifeless, sagging skin hung from her arms. I saw pointed, bony ribs so pronounced they were still visible through her baggy attire of nontoxic rags.

My legs were wobbly and weak, like tiny, brittle sticks. They could no longer hold me up. I weighed sixty pounds. I had subsisted exclusively on organic white rose potatoes for over two years! I rotated purified waters that were sent to me from all over the country. None, however, were pure enough for me to avoid a reaction.

My home was bare. The floor was plain, unpainted wood. The windows were kept tightly sealed for fear that any trace of toxins or fumes might enter. I could not venture outside of my home, and no one could enter.

I was thirty-five years old. My doctor told me that I would not make it to thirty-six. Seven years earlier, I had been diagnosed with lupus and environmental illness; both were deadly immune system dysfunctions. I began to experience the "universal reactor syndrome," one of the many symptoms of the disease. A universal reactor is a person who is allergic to all foods, chemicals and fumes — a person allergic to life itself.

For me, the most devastating part of it all was that I was allergic to people. It was impossible for me to be around other human beings! Everyone wore something that was toxic to me. With some it was perfume, deodorants, scented soaps, or hair spray. Others used dry cleaning fluids and fabric softeners. Even toothpastes and mouthwashes were intolerable; the slightest scent of any of it made me violently ill.

I had become so sensitive after my last medical treatment that I could not stand to be around anyone or anything that contained the slightest trace of chemicals or additives.

My problem with scented chemicals on bodies and clothing was just the beginning of my estrangement from the human race. My isolation was more personal than attire, much deeper in origin, much more complex. I reacted to the energy of people! I could feel their pain, their grief, their burdens, their bad days and concerns. I could not sit next to people without picking up their heartaches or deepest personal conflicts. I felt and reacted to their every emotion, every spirit, every thought — to any and all stimuli, whether they belonged to me or not.

I could no longer deal with this psychic interference; it was too bizarre. My rawness disconnected me from humanity. This was not a lifestyle I wanted to continue. I did not want to live another day without connection, companionship or hope.

## Been There, Done That

I had been resourceful in my attempts to recover my health. I tried all the international and local clinics, all the doctors,

3

dentists, and Indian chiefs (I say this literally), including acupuncturists, healers, homoeopaths, psychiatrists, psychologists, hypnotists and new age ministers. I had examined my feelings, released anger on the Gestalt chair and shared anonymously at twelve-step meetings. I no longer had codependency problems — I had no relationships. Not one source of human comfort.

I was willing to die just on the chance of fellowship in an afterlife. I still had faith in eternal life, but I had no faith to perpetuate the nightmare that had become my daily existence.

I wasn't anorexic. I didn't stop eating because I didn't like food. I was just afraid of the mental and physical reactions the food would bring. The reactions were so horrendous, so debilitating. I just could not recover from them anymore. There was nothing that would help me — no pain relief, no medication that could stop the reactions. I would go from anaphylactic shock to torturous muscle spasms — followed by chills and shaking, migraines, itching, head swellings and vomiting. After the disabling vomiting, there would be days of depression. The reactions were impossible for me to cope with any longer. They had totally traumatized me. They were so powerful that they intimidated me from eating any food, depriving me of any nutritional life force. I was actually starving. One by one I had relinquished foods that I reacted to on the prescribed allergy "elimination diet," until finally, there were no foods left; just my organic potatoes....

The allergic reactions were not just daytime attacks. They would also awaken me in the middle of the night, shaking me from my core to my extremities.

I would start off my attempt at sleep on my glass table, sans bedding materials, blankets and pillows. These normal comforts were usually made from synthetic materials. There was always something I was allergic to in the fabrics — the glue, the stitching, the dyes. Rounds of torment disturbed my sleep throughout the night. The first interruption of my sleep occurred on my antique, chemical-free glass table that had become my bed. After a couple of hours, I would be awakened by a shaking sensation deep in my core. It was as if I were vibrating! I would then move to my next location and hopefully pick up an undisturbed forty-five minutes of sleep on an old Salvation Army cot — one that had done its due diligence. It had been properly aired out for months; a precious hand-me-down from another environmentally ill insomniac.

Round three would take me to my faithful old wooden rocking chair, which was my only other piece of furniture. It was not good for my neck, but forty-five minutes of peace was worth neck pain. Every action had its own hostile punishment. I was looking forward to uninterrupted peace.

My decision was final. It was over. I had no place to go. I did not have anyone or anywhere to turn. I wanted out! My only concern was that I not suffer in dying. I constructed a plan.

I collected every pill I had saved over the years. I had enough saved to kill a sixty-pound person. I figured that the pills would take about fifteen minutes to render me unconscious....

## Something Primal

I felt confident and totally at peace with my decision to die — the kind of peace one feels when moving in a right direction. Then, strangely enough, I began to feel hungry! My stomach was empty and hollow; it wanted food! Usually my hunger was repressed by terror, but because I knew the threat of the allergic reactions would soon be over, I had the luxury of opening up to something natural and physical — food! For years I had forgotten I was starving! It didn't make any difference now. My reaction to this meal would be my last.

## Nothing Past Fifteen Minutes

I remember deciding to eat. Why not? What was the worst thing that could happen to me? Another bad fifteen minutes? Nothing past fifteen minutes could ever debilitate me again.

*I justified my fears of Hell by believing that I was in it.*

## The Last Supper

Jesus Christ Himself had a last supper when he decided to lay his life down. It was His choice. He was prophetically prepared. I enjoyed the last supper idea. I felt I was in good company.

I proceeded to order my last supper. I put on gloves to make the phone call. Everything had chemicals; everything was toxic on some level. I could feel the chemicals go through my skin.

I wore gloves to touch everything — to open an envelope, pay a bill. Without gloves, the glue and chemicals on all paper and materials would have seeped through my skin and into my bloodstream, creating more pain. Then there would be days of increased chemical sensitivities and unbearable chemical depression.

Carefully, I put on my 100% white cotton gloves to use the telephone. I dialed my 1950s round-faced rotary dial phone. It was the kind of phone you dialed manually, with big, metal circular holes for your fingers. There was a long waiting list for this type of phone. Many in the environmentally ill community would be grateful for such a find. It was simple, plain, big and black — an old table model sans the new (disturbing to some) touch-tone electronics.

I ordered my final meal. Even though making a phone call had potential harmful reactions, I knew that this would be my last call, and that encouraged me. I spoke to the restaurant employee, hoping to make my situation understood. I was embarrassed to have to explain in great detail how to leave the food I was ordering. I was aware that he probably thought I was insane.

I heard myself expressing ridiculous commands: "I will leave the money in a folder taped to the back door. I am here in the house, but I cannot open the door. Just leave the food outside on the step of the back door next to the garage. Don't park the truck in front of my house or in the driveway. I cannot tolerate any car fumes near my door when I open it. Please wrap the food in a double bag so fumes do not get on my food. I have allergies to petroleum."

Who was this creature ordering food like this? I wondered. Who was she?

I didn't want to live this "impostor's" life anymore!

This ordeal complete, I had survived the energy of another human being's voice and I was still functioning. My progress had not been thwarted. All I had to do was wait for the meal to arrive. When it came, I would not open the door for an additional fifteen minutes. I was afraid to risk the reaction of human contact. The many risks associated with opening my door could ruin my plan.

The only foods I had been able to eat up until this "Last Supper feast" were organic potatoes — the ones my ex-fiancé Tommy always left outside the back door. I would pick them up when no one was around. I would wait, of course, for the night air, wear three masks, quickly grab the bag and then run back in and slam the door shut.

I would make one last back-door pickup. I comforted my heart with that assurance.

This would be the first real meal I'd had in five years! Just the thought of eating a full dinner normally, carelessly, had my full attention.

I had to wait about forty minutes for the meal to arrive.

# The Goodbye Tape

I had no one to say goodbye to. I was totally disconnected from the world. I had only Tommy, who would drop off my organic white rose potatoes in the acceptable nontoxic manner. We could no longer interact; it was too painful for me. He was still available to me as a friend, as a potato dropper. He was living with another woman. Sometimes they would drop off the potatoes together. They both knew when I did not pick up my potatoes at the door that day that I was going to expedite my death. They did not try to stop me.

Tommy couldn't stand to see the torture. He later shared with me that he knew exactly what I was about to do and he didn't blame me. He agreed with my decision. There was, after all, no other way. All my previously close friends had suggested at one point or another that I end my life. It was the general consensus — what they would do in my situation. After all, they thought, what is the purpose of living like that?

## They Sensed My Decision

Tommy totally understood. We used to be able to speak to each other through my screen door until I became too sensitive even for that. Tommy got what was up when I didn't pick up the last potato shipment. He went home and cried all night in his new girlfriend Terri's arms.

As I waited for my last supper, I made a goodbye tape for him. I said goodbye to my last and only friend. I planned to leave my goodbye tape at our private hidden mailbox, outside the house near the garage door.

# Chapter 2

## Detox Gone Bad

When I first met Tommy, I was a completely different person, newly different, and not quite familiar with my new self. My new self had just emerged, having been created from a near-death experience, one that had produced in and of itself a change of plans, a life interrupted.

I had no spiritual inclinations when I left Los Angeles to spend my summer with a dear friend in Santa Barbara. I was there to have a good time, to rest, relax and enjoy a lovely summer vacation. I was generally a healthy person, although I had recently started having some allergic reactions to things — certain strong perfumes and a few airborne molds.

I decided to go on a health regimen to assuage these allergic irritations. An acquaintance referred me to a detoxification program that was being offered by Scientologists.

## The Scientologists

I was not prone to joining strange spiritual organizations. I was raised in New York City and grew up in a ghetto in the South Bronx. I wanted to accomplish something — to get somewhere different, somewhere kinder and gentler. I don't remember seeing any Scientologists canvassing the Bronx or seeing any Scientology buildings in the New York City ghettos.

My parents were not God-fearing folk. My mother was a Russian Jew and my dad a non-practicing Italian Catholic. There was not much spiritual orientation in my home. I did, however, have a privileged religious dichotomy. I was entitled to take every religious holiday in my elementary school. I could choose to be absent on all the Catholic and Jewish holidays. My parents thought it wise to expose me to all religions, thinking I would then be able to make my own decision ... so I experimented.

## Oy Vey

There was a season after my parents got divorced when my mother and I lived with my grandmother in the West Bronx, a mostly Jewish ghetto where I attended Hebrew school. My grandmother used to "kvell," a Jewish (Yiddish) word for rejoice, when I would read to her from the Hebrew newspaper. There was no God in any of it, no faith or any kind of spirituality.

In Jewish religious ghetto neighborhoods there is a cultural understanding. You don't have to "believe," but you do have to go through the motions. Mrs. Weisel, our next-door neighbor, was always aware of what we were doing. So were all the other neighbors. Everyone knew everyone else's slightest movement!

I would come home from school at about three-thirty every day, and as I walked up the three flights of stairs to our apartment, I would hear every apartment door open along the way, just enough for each tenant to peek out.

All the women and some of the men would sit outside in front of the building in little folding chairs. Everyone brought his or her own chair. It was a way to pass time — a social event. People would sit all day and most of the evening and watch all the folks come in and out of the building. They would comment on all the passersby. Gossiping was free entertainment in the Bronx. I am not talking about "Neighborhood Watch" programs; this was more intimate. It was more like "The Neighborhood Inquirer Association." They knew every date, every visitor a person ever had, and every purchase ever made. Everyone's personal business had to pass directly through the "chairs" in front of every building. I never felt it as hostile. It was just the way it was.

These were a lot of warm, loving people. Setting personal boundaries was not an issue; there were none.

We lit candles a lot. Every Jewish holiday had candles involved. You never wanted a neighbor to drop in and see that you did not light "the candles." As a family, we pretended to observe all the appropriate ritualistic religious behaviors. A relationship with God was never mentioned.

## Life in Queens, NY

My mother eventually remarried another non-practicing Italian Catholic, and we moved to Kew Gardens, Queens (somewhat of an upgrade). By then I was eight, and I was sent to study with a nun at a Catholic church in the new neighborhood. I had a wonderful connection with a lovely woman. She shared some workbooks and taught religious studies. I liked her a lot but still made no spiritual connection to God. That window rapidly closed after Lent.

Lent is the time when Catholics give something up, a sacrifice unto the Lord. I decided to cut my hair and nails. I don't know what I expected, but it was too big a sacrifice for a child who then suffered the repercussions of looking awful with short, ugly hair. It took me years to grow my long hair back. That turned me off to any further interest in Catholicism.

My mother was a dedicated atheist and did not encourage any additional religious teachings. My Lent despair was my final attempt to get spiritual input. I had seen no light! I had no further interest in finding God or religion, except for pursuing all the extra school holidays.

Eventually, my mother lost concern over which religion I was involved with or what school I attended. She had begun to drink heavily with my new stepfather. They were out most nights till five or six in the morning.

I saw no one at breakfast and no one at lunch. My mother usually met my stepfather downtown in the city for dinner. On rare occasions, they joined me for dinner (the only meal for which they were awake). These meals would be served in a drunken state at about ten or eleven at night. My main concern was that they not burn the kitchen down. This was not an unfounded fear, as the kitchen did go up in flames several times.

My stepfather's business was affiliated with the New York Mafia. I found him very hostile and intimidating. We made no real connection. He took pleasure in continually reminding me that I was another man's daughter. There was a song he liked to taunt me with whenever I crossed his path. It went like this: "From the wine came the grape and from the grape came the wine." For him it was a seed issue. I think that best sums up his old school Sicilian mentality.

The key to peace in my home was to stay out of everyone's way. The second important family rule was to leave for school very quietly in the morning so as not to disturb their drunken slumber. The third rule was to never tell anyone what was going on inside the home. This code of silence was imperative. *Omerta.*

## Purification

I share this background so that the reader might better understand why the "Scientology Cure" of putting two cans together to track past life dilemmas left something to be desired and explained as far as I was concerned. I had no interest in any of their modalities. However, there was a new program going around for allergies, a detoxification program performed in high-heat saunas. This detoxification program was being done in many doctors' offices as well as in the Scientology organization. They called this their "Purification Program."

## The Puriff

To a Scientologist, toxicity is the root of all evil. The Scientologists had recently gotten on the medical detox bandwagon and there was a Scientology detoxification center right in the middle of Santa Barbara. They generally used this treatment in their drug and alcohol program. I could write a book on the illusions of detoxification alone, and perhaps I have.

I was told that a person could detoxify from one week to thirty days and would be "free" when it was finished. I was told that the treatment would be complete when I no longer experienced symptoms of toxicity. Not only that, I could expect vibrant health and emotional well-being. All of my allergies would be gone, leaving a newer, cleaner, healthier, purified me. I didn't know any better. I did not investigate it at all. Had I done so, I would have discovered many lawsuits and a lot of damaged people. I had no idea that I was putting myself in jeopardy.

## Symptoms of Toxicity?

I was, after all, living in Southern California. If you are not, don't judge me too harshly. This was not a far-fetched idea in my community. I signed up for the program and followed the instructions closely.

I sat in a high-heat sauna for five hours a day for thirty-four days, waiting for the big release — the big nontoxic moment. I have since been informed that sitting in such high heat for an extended time is like being in a fire, and can destroy many organs in your body. I now understand that the hypothalamus and thyroid glands are the temperature controls of the body. The hypothalamus controls your brain; it is the first in command, followed by the pituitary and thyroid glands. On my post-Scientology quest for medical healing, I was often asked if I had been injured in a fire. Were they speaking symbolically? I've often wondered.

Every part of me wanted out. It was the middle of the summer in beautiful Santa Barbara, and I was sitting alone in a hot, uncomfortable sauna. But I was determined to finish the program and see the Scientologists' promises fulfilled. I believed that I was in integrity in my approach to the detoxification regime and would quit when I was authentically finished, even though my body, mind and soul were all screaming, "Get me out!" I put the Scientologists' expertise before my own feelings.

The believers of Scientology were guiding me! Believers! Believers in what? That was always the unanswered question. There was no God in Scientology. Their creator, founder and leader, L. Ron Hubbard, had died a mysterious death, his body never discovered. He had expired somewhere out in the ocean. There were lots of mysterious trips on elaborate yachts to which the upper-level Scientologists were privy. What went on during these journeys was never discussed. What exactly the Scientologists believed in I never found out — another unfulfilled promise. What was spiritual about that? I didn't yet comprehend that spirit can be other than the Spirit of God.

## Adding Toxins

I was hyped daily and given deadly toxic doses of multi-vitamins. I was taking close to a hundred supplements every day. My "toxicity" was actually being increased with unmonitored substances. I was not listening to my own inner voice. Instead, I was listening to the voices of crazy people. Every day they met with me and told me how great I was doing and how great I looked. They assured me that all the alleged toxins were coming out and that all was well. I was to be grateful for this blessing. These deadly poisons were finally being removed.

## I Was Finished

I waited patiently for the promised feelings that the program was "authentically finished"…but that "feeling good" signal never came. I remember the day that the program was over for me; I simply didn't have the physical strength to get back to the Scientology Center. I was totally drained, but I still wanted to force myself to go back. I knew that I had to get those last remaining toxins out! I was told that if I felt sick, I wasn't actually sick but was having a healing crisis from the outpouring of all the toxins. I could only imagine how sick they were making me internally if the toxins' exit could be so debilitating! That was their last week's story when I was still ambulatory, when all my friends had warned me, when it was clear to all that I was having a health crisis, not a healing crisis!

I was having a lapse of consciousness, a mind crisis, being deceived by a cult. Even my non-spiritual friends could see that. It was clear to everyone that my health was being destroyed by an insane detoxification regimen under the guise of what the Scientologists called their "Purification Program."

## My Last Day

I was told to continue with the program. They had an explanation as to why I was feeling so ill: repressed toxins were working their way out. I was threatened enough by this "don't get stuck in the middle" plea to continue with the sauna. That last day, even though I felt so sick, I still wanted to push further and go back to the Center.

Maybe this would be it — a final release, my completion followed by my reward. I was clinging to that hope for my miracle. Perhaps the promise of freedom would be revealed on that last day!

## A Walking Psychic Wound

I crawled into my bathroom to take my shower and return to the Center. I put the light on and reacted to it. I reacted to a light bulb! How was that possible?

Suddenly I was in another realm. My diagnosis had changed. This was no longer just a case of a few allergies! I was psychically possessed.

I had a girlfriend who was on vacation in Hawaii. I heard and felt her thoughts. I called her to confirm my experiences, and she listened to my suspicions. I knew her thoughts, her feelings and her current situation! I was raw. I was totally opened, totally sensitized to everything. I was a walking psychic wound. I had never been mentally sensitive or psychic. I had never believed in or spoken with psychics. I had no interest in them. Now I knew why; this was hell on earth!

## I Was in Another World

All I knew was that my current reality had changed. I became the most sensitive person on this planet, bar none. No one was in my league. My roommate Annie came home that day and saw me lying down exhausted. She was not a big Scientology fan to begin with, but she was shocked to see me that weakened.

"What happened to you?" Annie asked. "You look worse today than I've ever seen you look. Don't go back there any more, Juliana. Stay away from them. They are evil!"

When I told Annie that I had reacted to the light in our bathroom she was aghast. What I didn't tell her was that I was reacting to her also! I reacted to her feelings, her words, her fears, and her thoughts. I was so opened up, so raw, that I reacted to everything.

# I Call for Help

I called the Scientologists that day and explained my situation. I let them know, "I will not be coming back." I was allergic to everything on Earth. Something strange had happened to me in the purification program. I was overly purified! I couldn't digest food. I was reacting to my bed; I couldn't lie down on my mattress. I was reacting to my roommate's thought forms. I was so pure that everything was toxic to me. I had lost my tolerance for life.

# They Are Clueless

The Scientologists have no clue. They had never seen this type of response before, or so they claimed. After their initial defensiveness and denial, the Scientologists made a comeback. They came up with a new theory. They wanted to "can" me.

# The Magic Wand of the Scientologists

The "cans" are the Scientologists' method of healing — their crystals, their magic wand. As far as the Scientologists are concerned, the "cans" are all that one needs. They would solve my problem!

However, there would be a delay; the "can" barometer suggested that my system was too low to proceed. I did not have enough vitamin B in my system for the can healing to begin! The cylinders required certain health standards. They declined my need!

The Scientologists were waiting for a green light from the "cans" themselves, which were allegedly able to discern human vitamin levels, especially vitamin B. Where was my vitamin B? Had I not been ingesting over 2,000 milligrams of this vitamin daily on their purification program?

The Scientologists apparently knew exactly what my real problem was. Interpreted in "can" lingo, it was simply this: I had gotten sidetracked, stuck between lives. I was in a conflict of lifetimes! These past life conflicts, not karma, exactly, but a "hook," a "trigger" from a previous moment in another time, another life, another situation, were creating havoc in my current life. My perfect detoxification and release of all unnatural toxins had been interrupted by a past life mishap. The "cans," fortunately, had the knowledge to correct this type of interference and could intervene on my behalf.

"What is in the cans," you must be thinking, "to have such power?" They were empty. They were not specially made, just aluminum soup cans. I still haven't gotten an answer as to the reason for their supernatural power.

A string attached the two aluminum cylinders to each other. It was nothing special … just two cans attached to plain old string; this would be my healer and track my real problem, which had absolutely nothing to do with the high heat abuse I had just experienced, according to the Scientologists.

That's all the Scientologists had to offer! I was reacting to thoughts, lights, friends, and my bed (that had suddenly changed to 100% cotton futon). They offered nothing except two cans on a string, which they claimed had the potential to change lives.

Not mine, however. Not yet. I was on my own, confused and desperate.

I had to seek other avenues of help. I canned the Scientologists. They were grateful to avoid me. They did their best to run from me, fearing a lawsuit. I was too sick to sue. I prayed to God.

# Chapter 3

## Life Post "Cans"

I was invited to do a meditation by one of the neighbors who noticed my new sensitivity. She interpreted my problem as one she had experienced herself: chronic fatigue syndrome and Candida (at least that was an impression in current time and in this life). She had compassion for my strange plight. I decided to go to the meditation. I divorced myself from all "can" mentalities and moved on. I hoped that this might be God's new plan.

## Watch and Pray

*Matthew 26:41: "Watch and pray, that ye enter not into temptation: the spirit indeed is willing, but the flesh is weak."*

The minister was a lovely young Christian woman who held meditations in her home. They were very intimate, very nurturing. They weren't selling anything — no programs, no detox. They believed in God. It wasn't a mystery. They stated it openly. I was grateful to be there.

Everyone was quite charming and kind. I followed and did the meditation and prayers. I felt great the next day and decided to do another prayer and meditation at home on my own. I found I could "still" my mind quite easily, and my body was healing rapidly. I made a connection within, and was now being led to a more personal meditation, one led by the spirit — the Spirit of God. With a few short practices, I had the power to still my entire mind!

I still couldn't look at a pill of any kind. The overdose of vitamins from the Scientology detoxification had permeated my system, and my digestive system was shot. However, I began making a remarkable comeback. I continued doing my fifteen-minute-a-day meditation. My mind started to become still, as if it were on automatic pilot. I was now doing two fifteen-minute-a-day meditations. My life was changing. I was leaving the psychic time zone and entering into the peace of God!

My meditation was simple. I would surrender all my thoughts, one by one, and then I would feel connected to God. When my meditation was complete, my moment would be retrieved. I would return to my flow — my thoughts stopped, my peace restored.

God was slowing me down. If I wanted to connect to God and feel His Presence, all I had to do was slow down my thoughts. When my mind was slowed down, I had peace and could be led by the Holy Spirit. God had His own time! Today I would call that time slot the Dispensation of Grace.

We all know the blue car phenomena. When you have one you notice one. And suddenly the entire world had Christ, perfect peace and love. My world had changed.

*Matthew 5:9: "Blessed are the peacemakers;*
*for they shall be called the children of God."*

## Perceptions of Grace

I had perfect peace and perfect love. I was meeting the most interesting people. My life had become a constant parade of sincere seekers and great friends that wanted to have a good time.

*John 14:27: "Peace I leave with you, my peace I give unto you."*

## The Scientologists Disappeared

The Scientologists suddenly, magically disappeared. They were in a different time zone. They were still working it out, still trying to get there via the sauna and the "cans." Grace was of no interest to them.

## The Power of Grace

The power of grace, I was discovering, could take a person into another dimension. I had been transformed — from almost dying from spiritual oppression to being a loving vessel for Christ. Grace had the power to regenerate a spirit and sanctify a soul. Grace could work without striving, without people, doctrine or dogma. Grace was my key to the Kingdom of God, and with this grace all the fruit of the spirit would flow through me.

*Ephesians 2:5: "Even when we were dead in sins, hath quickened us together with Christ (by grace ye are saved)."*

I was being quickened together with the Spirit of Christ.

Even as we are regenerating daily (growing and advancing in the Spirit), we are able to have full power over our flesh. Spiritual dominion is activated by faith, not by personal progress. Your dominion is your inherited power as a child of God on this earth. You don't get more for being better, or less for being worse.

Your dominion has nothing to do with your sex life or how much you tithe or help others.

Your dominion is established by your faith in the finished work of the Cross of Calvary.

*Ephesians 2:8: "For by grace are ye saved through faith; and that not of yourselves: it is the gift of God."*

21

# Chapter 4

## Walking with God

Walking with God was new to me, and I had never been happier! I guess I had never known happiness before, not like this — total peace, love and joy. The Holy Spirit led me everywhere I went. I was always, quite naturally, in the right place at the right time.

I was blessed everywhere. People felt me and I felt them. I had had no idea how privileged a place this was! I was resonating in a divine vibration, attracting like-minded souls. I clearly saw that everybody was exactly where he or she was supposed to be without religiosity, dogma or judgment. God was in control.

There was so much love in the world. My world had become a very blessed place. Synchronicity surrounded me, and I was having a grand time.

*Galatians 5:22: "But the fruit of the spirit is love,*
*joy, peace, longsuffering, gentleness, goodness, faith."*

## Slow Time

I upped my two fifteen-minute meditations to three fifteen-minute sessions a day. With three daily meditations, I began to connect very deeply from my center and very deeply to others with whom I resonated. It was as if we were able to identify each other — a Holy Spirit vibe. There was something in the energy, a peace; something in the eyes, a wisdom, a depth, a softness and an openness. It seemed the slower the time, the more open the heart!

This was a time to be open, to feel deeply, to tarry and yield unto the Lord. It was a time of willingness to be available to receive what was going on with an expectation of faith. What I was calling "slow time" was just pure spirit. Surrendering my thoughts to God's "slow time" exchanged my thoughts for the Mind of Christ! My carnal mind was bowing to the supremacy of God's Kingdom power.

## The Kingdom of God

When my mind was slowed down, I was deepened. It was as if I were standing two feet behind myself, behind my own heart, hidden deep within myself and hidden in Christ. My very breath would be deepened, as if I were experiencing the breath of God Himself! I was starting to hear the voice of God. My path was coming to me.

I had been spiritually chosen to be on my path. I was definitely following Christ. Being Jewish on my mom's side made Christianity not my natural inclination. It was at first even difficult to say the "J" word.

*Matthew 6:33: "Seek ye first the kingdom*
*of God and all else will be added unto you."*

## Reverend Kiki Calls It Guidance

I was beginning to get what Rev. Kiki, my minister friend, called guidance. "Guidance," Rev. Kiki would explain, "is when you hear from God; then you can be led."

## I See Christ in All

I was convinced that all meditators, every spiritual being, every person who had prayed a prayer was in paradise and walked with God. I saw God in everyone. I had been so opened up in the sauna, purified to rawness.

23

I could feel what was left inside a human being when all the walls and defenses were removed! Underneath it all, without the defenses and barriers of life, was the perfect love of God and the perceptions of Christ. I realized that this is who we really are.

I was not a seeker when I began this journey. I knew very little. My spiritual training was nonexistent. My only safety in this new realm, my only protection, was in being led. I had to be led; everything was about cautiously surrendering to the leading of God.

> *Galatians 5:17: "For the flesh lusteth against the Spirit, and the Spirit against the flesh: and these are contrary the one to the other: so that ye cannot do the things that ye would."*

> *Galatians 5:18: "But if ye be led of the Spirit, ye are not under the law."*

## Be as a Butterfly

> *Galatians 5:1: "Stand fast therefore in the liberty wherewith Christ hath made us free, and be not entangled again with the yoke of bondage."*

I was hearing from God, and His instructions were clear. He was telling me, *"Stay free, be as a butterfly; love all people the same. Do not be a respecter of persons. Do not get attached, and do not get entangled!"*

I had no idea how important that revelation was! I had no idea that that statement was life and death! I did not know this word was given to me because I was not prepared to take on the barrage of familiar spirits that would await a newly awakened soul.

Sometimes God will take you the long way because He knows exactly what you need to do to strengthen. The Holy Spirit told me to connect and move on. I was told to expand who I am, not get stuck anywhere, not be brought down. And, like a butterfly, enjoy a season of flying solo.

I loved everyone equally. I perceived everyone as being perfect, working out his or her soul's path, moving ahead in his or her personal purpose. My ability to hear the thoughts of others and the intrusive psychic realm was being absorbed by the new, larger opening of my heart. My mind was yielding to my connection with God. I was free!

> *Philippians 2:2: "Fulfill ye my joy, that ye be likeminded, having the same love, being of one accord, of one mind."*

## An Open Heart

The opening of my heart and the regeneration of my spirit were greater than the influence of the carnal mind. I was in grace. I was walking around in the highest consciousness I had ever experienced. All of my perceptions had changed!

> *Ezekiel 36:26: "A new heart also will I give you, and a new spirit will I put within you: and I will take away the stony heart out of your flesh, and I will give you an heart of flesh."*

# Chapter 5

## Spiritual Warfare

I had no clue that I had entered into a spiritual war zone. No idea that I would be challenged. Or that I would have to hold onto this place.

I had no knowledge of any of this — just the place, the spot. I was deep in His Kingdom. It was mine. Why would I doubt my capacity to keep my heart free? I had security in high places. I was living the new and better me.

> Matthew 11:12: "And from the days of John
> the Baptist until now the kingdom of heaven
> suffereth violence, and the violent take it by force."

## Living Again

I was up and living again. Out and about, my roommate Annie and I would go out dancing and have fun. We went to all the local Santa Barbara events. I enjoyed meeting new people and was confident that all was well.

I no longer had any negative and critical judgments about others. I accepted everyone with an open heart, mind, and unconditional love. I was not interested in romance at this time; I was nurturing my Holy relationship. I did have some interesting characters pursuing me, but I sensed that the season wasn't right.

There were other reasons that I was being pursued. There were spiritual challenges that I was not aware of at all. They were the reason for God's warning words to "stay free ... don't get involved ... be as a butterfly."

*2 Timothy 1:13: "Hold fast the form of sound words, which
thou hast heard of me, in faith and love which is in Christ Jesus."*

## Hid in Christ

I thought the revelation God had imparted to my spirit was
delightful! Be as a butterfly! Be free! How charming! How liber-
ating!

Had I been a more advanced student of the Spirit, I would
have rapidly replied, "Yes, Lord, I will stay hidden in you. I will
be led. Lead me, Jesus, in your righteousness. Stay close till I am
standing separate from my old nature, from my generational
past, till my life is dead in you."

If I were going to keep my healing, I would have to remain
as "me," the new me, the spirit woman. I would have to hang
on the hem of His garment for a while.

I was a baby. I could not crawl on my own yet — walking
separately from Jesus was unthinkable! I was newly separated
from my total past and living the "new creature in Christ" reality.
I would have to learn to stand against my generational past, and
to be able recognize emotions and thoughts that did not belong
to me!

*Psalm 27:5: "For in the time of trouble he shall hide
me in his pavilion: in the secret of his tabernacle
shall he hide me; and he shall set me upon a rock."*

## A New Creature

My relationships would all have to line up with the purpose
of God. The purpose of God would keep me sanctified while I
strengthened. I did not have any unusual cosmic relationship
problems prior to this time.

My problems were like those of most people — your aver-
age, garden-variety neurotic relationship dilemmas of the twenti-
eth century kind. I had never experienced any strange or

supernaturally created evil devised to take me down and pull me out of grace! I didn't understand or believe that those types of problems existed. I thought that all of the strange and unusual happenings had ended when I left the Scientologists and connected to God.

However, I had been deliberately broken down in the "puriff" program; this had opened doors to spiritual attacks, oppositions that I was unable to even perceive, let alone handle. My defenses had been weakened on many levels. God's purpose had been temporarily thwarted.

*Ephesians 1:11: "In whom also we have obtained an inheritance, being predestinated according to the purpose of him who worketh all things after the council of his own will."*

## Wolves in Sheep's Clothing

One of my pursuers at this time was a very unusual but wholesome-appearing character. He was a little more aggressive than the rest, the type of man who knew how to push himself ahead in a line. He was an unusual combination of sincerity and perseverance.

I am talking about the same man who would eventually drop my potatoes off at death's door.

*2 Corinthians 11:14: "And no marvel; for Satan himself is transformed into an angel of light."*

## The Potato Man

Tommy had become infatuated with me. He was new in town, having just arrived from Kenya, where he had had to leave his home and business due to a political upheaval. His life had been threatened, and he was stressed and unsettled. He was looking for connection, friendship, romance and ground. In short, he was lonely.

I was not looking for any of these things or feeling needy. I was glad to be alive! I was being the butterfly. I was having fun! My life was full, purposeful, and peaceful.

I expressed my position to Tommy. I loved him as much as anyone else, as a brother, but I didn't want to get romantically involved. I offered a platonic friendship. He accepted, saying, "I'll take anything I can get." He would be delighted to be my friend.

We were in very different places in our lives. I was a woman separating myself from my old ways, beginning to connect from a deep place within my own being, my center.

He was a man who drove into a conservative town in a big red Porsche. He was not pretentious, just flamboyant and self-conscious. On paper, my friend Tommy was the perfect man. He was thirty-four years old, a self-made millionaire. If I had to sum Tommy up in one word, I would say tenacious. His intelligence was based on his tenacity. He didn't need creative genius to make things happen. He knew how to aggress his way to the top.

Tommy had never married and had the perfect Ivy League education. He loved and wanted children, and he was probably the most loyal man on the planet. He was attractive — tall, thin and regal, with beautiful dark hair, shiny green eyes — and charming in a boyish way.

*Proverbs 4:23: "Keep thy heart with all
diligence; for out of it are the issues of life."*

## Carnal Mind Control

There was one unusual personality trait that I had overlooked. He was too easily distracted in conversation. He had a limited focus, the type of person who, when you are saying something, is looking at the wall thinking something else, not responsive in the moment. His response was in another zone, too late, on the wrong topic or with an inappropriate segue. His conversation didn't connect with my heart!

There is a name for this behavior: attention deficit syndrome. He couldn't hold a moment. "Momentus interruptus," I like to call it. A mind gone wild. Carnal mind in control!

Tommy was not a "slow time" candidate. He was on fast time — talking fast, babbling, always in a hurry, always running somewhere. He was very distracting. He was not a grounded, centered-in-Christ kind of man! He was not God's choice for me.

His energy would eventually oppose my peace. I did not know that another human being's energy could oppose my peace! I had no knowledge of principalities and spiritual wickedness manipulating and moving through people. I didn't realize that his continuous lack of focus would affect my ability to have an open heart. I didn't understand how to protect my heart. Nor did I know it was necessary. I was unaware that this lack of substantial connection or authentic attention would wear me down.

*Romans 8:7: "For the carnal mind is enmity against God:*
*for it is not subject to the law of God, neither indeed can it be."*

## The Impostor

I went into denial. I was unable to properly identify the impossibility of the connection. My old nature, the "impostor" of my newly regenerated spirit woman, did not want to admit that Tommy and I were not compatible, that we were on different planets, and that we had totally different destinies. Somehow my old nature felt a responsibility toward this man.

I was not in romantic love with him. He had declared his love for me, which had somehow, in my generational past, triggered an ungodly loyalty and responsibility for his happiness! *The "impostor's" attraction to the law via generational guilt reared its ugly head!*

*Romans 8:12: "Therefore, brethren, we are*
*debtors, not to the flesh, to live after the flesh."*

## What I Didn't Know

I didn't know that I could lose slow time. I thought that it was mine, that it came with the new me. I didn't know that it was up for grabs. I didn't know that if I lost my peace, I would also lose the slowing down of my thoughts, and I would not be able to connect to God. I didn't know that it was possible to lose the entire healing that I had been so blessed with after the "purification program." I had no idea that I could go back to that raw state. I didn't even suspect that I was at risk.

I knew that I was in "slow time," God's time, in His Grace, and in His Kingdom. I felt no insecurity at all. For the first time in my life, I felt absolute confidence, not a tinge of paranoia. I thought that I was the messenger of peace, that I could help Tommy. I had no idea that, at this time, I couldn't survive his speeded-up energy. My concern and obsession was to help and heal "poor Tommy."

*Hosea 4:6: "My people are destroyed for lack of knowledge ..."*

## More Stuff I Didn't Know

What I didn't know was that "perfect love" cast out fear. Perfect love was not romantic love — it was the love of God. God's love responded with faith and peace. It was unconditional.

> *1 John 4:18: "There is no fear in love; but*
> *perfect love casteth out fear: because fear hath*
> *torment. He that feareth is not made perfect in love."*

I didn't know that perfect love would be challenged, refined and tried by fire. Perfect love would have to contain a balance of love and authority to be able to withstand that which was unlike itself. Perfect love would initiate a war of temptations. It was not a signed, sealed and delivered deal. Just as it had been granted in peace, it could disappear in stress.

How do you get something back that you did nothing to acquire in the first place? I would not be able to retrace my steps. I could not do one hundred things right to get it back. I would surely try, though, and that would be another stumbling block to grace itself — the biggest one of them all.

> *Romans 9:32: "Wherefore? Because they sought it*
> *not by faith, but as were by the works of the law.*
> *For they stumbled at that stumbling stone."*

## I Didn't Know the Power of Purpose

I didn't know that I had survived the Scientology ordeal due to a predestined before-the-foundation-of-time purpose in God.

My spirit had a purpose. It was not the prayer or meditations or Reverend Kiki's teachings. It was My Divine Purpose. My purpose in God had the power to keep me alive and to raise me from the dead. *The purpose of God is the strongest force on this earth and can heal or remove anything in its way.*

I didn't know that leaving God's purpose was the creator of all disharmony, of all illness on earth, and that my spirit would collapse. The spirit is alive through righteousness, and righteousness has God's purpose in mind.

*Romans 8:10: "The Spirit is life because of righteousness."*

# Say What?

Righteousness is simply the obedient action of God's purpose. I didn't know that I had a purpose (not to help another, not to rescue the world, not codependency) but a real purpose — a personal destiny. No one ever had mentioned personal spiritual purpose to me.

I'd heard talk of love, tithing, sermons on sin and healing. I never heard anyone mention that if you want to stay alive and prosper on this earth, you had better get hold of God's purpose in your life. God's purpose will solve all of your problems. The purpose of God has within itself enough fuel, enough resurrection power, to move you through any illness, any trauma or any problem on earth. No one told me that God would back His purpose. Yes, Jesus loves me, but predestined purpose had favor.

*Ephesians 1:9: "Having made known unto us the mystery of His will, according to his good pleasure which he hath purposed in Himself."*

# Chapter 6

## The Opposition Will Twist Predestined Purpose

I am not talking about serving God. We all know that God uses different people in different ministries and different vocations. Everyone serves God in their own special way with their own special gifts. For some people, there is sometimes an additional ministry purpose (this should not negate a personal purpose).

*Ecclesiastes 3:1: "To everything there is a season,
and a time to every purpose unto heaven."*

*Ecclesiastes 3:11: "He hath made everything beautiful in his time,
also he hath set the world in their heart, so that no man can find
out the work that God maketh from the beginning to the end."*

## Predestined Purpose

There is another purpose, a very personal purpose, that your individual spirit came to achieve. This purpose is transformational. It is a development of your spiritual qualities, attributes and authority! This purpose serves to develop and empower you as a separate and complete entity. This purpose keeps you sanctified and in control over the wiles of the impostor (the counterfeit of your true identity). This personal purpose quickens you in life! The opposition to your purpose, the old nature, will attempt to get you off the purpose track. If you are led away from purpose (the old nature's constant focus and goal), you will be powerless.

No matter how much you pray, read the Bible or do good works, *if you are not in your personal purpose, you will have difficulty being upheld. You will not get your heart to work for you. All the powerful forces of life will be blocked from your daily experiences.*

Maybe once in awhile you will get some joy, but generally speaking, you are pushing against the wind, fighting an uphill battle, not living high in the Lord. Life becomes a continuous hardship, not a flow of grace. And your enemy, the old nature, will try to deceive you into religious thinking.

A big con of the law of sin and death is to use the spirit of condemnation to deceive you into believing you are here to do good works, that your purpose has to do with someone else's needs. This "enmity" of God will try to create a codependent purpose that is outside of your self and your eternal orders. It will be a "look good purpose," an inauthentic purpose, to keep you out of the Kingdom of God and out of your joy. It is really the purpose of guilt to keep you in bondage! If you wake up every day in joy, you are in purpose.

## Your Purpose Is About You!

I am talking about a lifelong purpose here, the purpose of the individual spirit and the opportunity for personal growth. Your spirit is here to grow, to climb the ladder of enlightenment! A spirit that accomplishes its purpose can go home fulfilled and satisfied. A spirit that has lived an oppressed life far from its purpose is miserable. It is forced into living a fruitless life. It may look like a blessed and good life to the casual observer, *but if the spirit is in a purposeless life, there is misery, illness and discontent.*

You could be serving the Lord, have a huge and successful ministry and be out of this very personal purpose. This personal purpose may not look Godly, it might even sometimes look ridiculous. This purpose is between you and the Lord. Do not be talked out of it; it has the power to keep you in divine health and joy!

> *Romans 8:30: "Moreover, whom he did predestinate, them also he called, and whom he called, them he also justified, and whom he justified, them he also glorified."*

## What Is Depression?

Today I am grateful to know what depression is. When I am feeling grief, it is a sign to me, an omen. It is a word from the Lord that I am moving in a direction far from my purpose. It is an indication that I have been led away by deception. I have lost my way. I am about to be disempowered! Today, it is a gift to know that I can turn myself around, take authority over error and do something else. The feeling of grief or depression is actually the old nature throwing you off track and then thinking its thoughts in your mind!

God does not dump us because we miss a mark. The old nature takes advantage of us being deceived and misled and uses that opportune moment to punish and condemn us.

Grief is an emotional response to the misadventure created by the law of sin and death itself. It opposes the forgiveness and freedom of Christ and His Perfect Law of Liberty. You were misled; simply let go of all your thoughts and walk into the new moment by faith. Call a new moment in God!

> *2 Corinthians 3:17: "Now the Lord is that Spirit: and where the Spirit of the Lord is, there is liberty."*

A purposeless and powerless life creates depression. It is a life not led by God. It is that simple! The emotion of grief is a sign of *victimization*, authority relinquished and deception spoken, heard and received. You know when you are entering into God's purpose and His will by the amazing peace.

## A Seed War

Like most people that are in a spiritual battle, I didn't see its roots. I did not know about the war between the flesh and the spirit, the new creature versus the old.

*Galatians 5:17: "For the flesh sets its desire against the spirit, and the spirit against the flesh."*

I didn't know who I was. I didn't know that my true seed was the seed of Christ, the seed of righteousness, and that this seed was sown in purpose. In order to have this seed expand and give me life, I would have to water it with pure, unadulterated purpose.

*Galatians 3:16: "Now to Abraham and his seed were the promises made. He hath not said, And to seeds, as of many, but as of one, And to thy seed, which is Christ."*

I would have to live my essence, the spirit woman, in every facet of my life. My real life, my life in Christ, would be happy and empowered only when in His Purpose. If I were to win the battle between the flesh and the spirit, purpose would have to be fulfilled. Any step towards purpose would be upheld and honored; my spirit would rise up and my heart would open. I would rejoice. Any step away from purpose would do the exact opposite. My spirit would grieve, my heart would shut down and my life force would be quenched!

*1 Thessalonians 5:19: "Quench not the spirit."*

## Keep Your Eyes on Purpose!

One thing you never want to do in life is negate God's purpose. You are here for a reason, a purpose. You have a mission. You and your mission are very important to God. Being "you" is your best defense.

> *2 Timothy 1:9: "Who hath saved us and called*
> *us with a holy calling, not according to our works,*
> *but according to his own purpose and grace, which*
> *was given us in Christ Jesus before the world began."*

## Faith Worketh by Love

I had perfect love for Tommy and everyone else. Perfect love is not a respecter of persons, and this type of love would not contradict my purpose.

> *Acts 10:34: "God is no respecter of persons."*

Codependent love, and its illusion of romantic love, brings with it its carnal capacity to pull one out of the spirit and harden your heart. This can be very oppressive. Mortal or carnal love is the quickest way to lose your separation from your inner impostor on this earth. There is no truth in it.

I had been walking in perfect love, but I had not yet developed perfect authority. I had not yet developed any authority. I didn't even have personal power. I was naive in my battle.

> *Galatians 5:6: "For in Christ Jesus neither circumcision availeth*
> *anything, nor uncircumcision, but faith which worketh by love."*

## How I Was Seeing It (Or How I Wasn't Seeing It)

I felt sorry for Tommy. He seemed like a lost soul. He was like a big dog that was protective and loyal and wanted to be in the middle of everything. I nicknamed him Big Dog. It stuck.

> *Luke 6:39: "And he spake a parable*
> *unto them, can the blind lead the blind?"*

## What's Love Got to Do with It?
## (Tina Really Did Know, Didn't She?)

I told Big Dog over and over what I needed to do for myself. I was clear about what I wanted at that time in my life. I wanted and needed peace. I needed to be left alone to continue to regain my health and pursue my daily meditations. I expressed to Tommy that I needed time for prayer to hold my newly gained center and relationship with God.

I continually expressed this boundary to him. I told him I needed space. My words were spoken to help him understand, not to protect me. I was taking care of him!

## Guilt

*Sin consciousness (guilt) always tries to force you to take care of your enemy and help the opposition.* It is a manipulation of evil, a ploy to take one out of their purpose. When one has no purpose, one has no power. Guilt wants you to be externally focused, to further keep you unaware of its thinking process. It is plotting to keep you in denial and self-justification, to arrest your moving ahead in your purpose.

Instead of moving ahead, you will be trying to fix your problems that are being created deliberately to keep you off the purpose empowerment trail. After a few good distractions, you might be deceived into a lot of time-consuming drama and pain!

Your problems are not what they appear to be. They are perceptual errors of inherited generational unconsciousness. Your problems can only be solved by the restoration of your righteousness consciousness. The resolution of all your problems is a rapid return to your proper identity.

*Romans 6:6: "Knowing this, that our old man is crucified with him, that the body of sin might be destroyed, that henceforth we should not serve sin."*

## My Words Were Not Honored

Tommy ignored my verbal request for boundary. I was too impressed with his utter devotion to me and had too much pity (guilt) for his neediness to back my words up with a good kick in the butt or a final good-bye. I was unable to make my needs heard or obeyed. He chose to expedite his plan. He moved into one of the units in my condo complex.

I didn't see it! I would have needed to perceive it with a spiritual consciousness that I had not yet developed. He was gaining territory, moving in closer to his target, and I was acquiescing and losing ground! I didn't acknowledge it even to myself! I didn't know I was in a battle for my spiritual life! I had no inclination that he was opposing my identity, my very existence!

Tommy's great gift was that he knew how to take care of himself. He was in control. He could manipulate and delegate guilt like a commanding officer of sin consciousness itself. I found myself thinking, *Poor Tommy. He is alone and needs to get involved with a new job and new friends.*

"Poor Tommy" would knock on my door daily, always at the perfect moment that would destroy my peace. These interruptions at ungodly times occurred so often that soon his phone calls could be perceived in my heart and in my stomach. The ring of the phone that identified him would go right through me. It felt as if someone were actually throwing a dart or drilling a hole in my gut. His very energy became an armed weapon of demonic spiritual warfare.

Had he been an alcoholic, a drug addict, a woman beater, an obviously abusive man, I could have recognized it. I was no match! I was blinded by guilt.

*Deuteronomy 19:13: "Thine eye shall not pity him, but thou shalt put away the guilt of innocent blood from Israel."*

## The Agenda of Codependency

Tommy's interest in or conscious understanding of my center, my needs, was minimal. He was interested in his goal. He had found the dream girl and he could now get on with his plan, his agenda! He wanted to end his loneliness, get married, have children, raise a family and have lots of friends. It is very seductive to be adored.

Guilt had a mesmerizing power to make me feel "wrong" for not returning this idyllic love. The truth in my heart was clear; my newly found center was much more important than Tommy or any other man. I wasn't in love with him romantically. This challenge was not about unrequited love.

The test was about taking care of me, about my not giving up my space to someone else. I couldn't see it. Was it wrong to have a good man devoted to me? Should I instead find myself a loser, a verbally abusive person, or a man who would be unfaithful? What was wrong with this picture? I was unable to identify or define the spiritual abuse of someone who had no regard for my spirit, my purpose or my relationship with God.

I was like the proverbial leaf at sea, tossed about by the waves of false doctrines and consumed by inherited generational guilt.

*Matthew 7:15: "Beware of false prophets, which come to you in sheep's clothing, but inwardly they are ravening wolves."*

## The White Picket Fence

The illusion of romance is strong in our earthly consciousness. This illusion has been deeply ingrained in our carnal nature. It has been handed down throughout the generations and imparted to us on many different levels. We have been programmed that this love can be obtained through our carnal natures and is necessary to our carnal selves.

This belief is inundated deep in a woman's consciousness. We learned early on from our mothers that no compromise is too great to get this prize! The ultimate goal for a woman is to fall in love, marry, have children and obtain the white picket fence! Only then do we have security and peace, according to this deception.

Tommy, my aggressive friend, was the personification of the white picket fence. I did not misread him! He was sincere. He was what he represented himself to be.

> *Jeremiah 16:19: "Surely our fathers have inherited lies, vanity, and things wherein there is no profit."*

# Chapter 7

## Must Have Been the Wrong Time

Tommy and I had different destinies. My consciousness had recently been elevated beyond the carnal mind control programming and the illusions of carnal love. This mentality would not serve me in my new purposes! The white picket fence had become undesirable to me. My spirit knew way beyond my capacity to understand that this was a set-up for me. This inner battle was unrecognizable to me.

I did know in my heart when I really did not want to see him. I could feel it, but I didn't trust my own desire to renounce an old script. He would constantly just drop by and knock on my door. "Juliana, come out and play. I am lonely. Just come out for a moment, for a lunch, a movie or a dinner, a walk!"

I didn't feel or hear my own heart that was enraged at his insensitivity and aggression. My life force was being quenched.

*Ecclesiastes 7:7: "Surely oppression maketh a wise man mad ..."*

## My Spirit Knew How to Handle It

*1 Corinthians 2:10: "But God hath revealed them unto us by his Spirit: for the Spirit searcheth all things, yea, the deep things of God."*

My spirit knew how to take care of me: "Tommy, you are disturbing my peace, how dare you! You did this yesterday, you did this today, and if you ever do this again, you will have to get out of the line of fire. I am so entangled in your agenda, I can no longer see straight. My sleep is interrupted and I can't digest my food. You are not respecting my boundaries. Get thee hence, mister!"

I didn't feel the rage. I didn't feel the truth. My denial oppressed my spirit and rendered my only defense ineffective! I was busy being considerate to Tommy. After all, he loved me and wanted a white picket fence future with me.

## Numbed by Guilt

My generational nature and the guilt therein were too strong. I was programmed to stand by my man. Even if I didn't want him, he was still a man. What I wanted, what my heart was screaming for, had nothing to do with it. I was conditioned to pay little attention to my own desires and inner voice. My soul was to be negotiated by the opposite sex.

*Ezekiel 20:18: "But I said unto the children in the wilderness, Walk ye not in the statutes of your fathers, neither observe their judgments, nor defile yourself with their idols."*

## Sin Consciousness Programming (Total Unconsciousness)

The voice of condemnation and the sin consciousness therein would have you believe that if an unworthy creature such as yourself has the good fortune to be offered a "white picket fence," you should be grateful and jump at the chance of this promise of security — immediately letting go of any plans, ideas, friends, aspirations, dreams or innate talents. In this case, my life's purpose and destiny in Christ were the issue, and they were being rapidly oppressed.

Guilt and condemnation had attacked and shut down my heart. My fire was going out rapidly, almost extinguished. I became totally disconnected from my righteous indignation. I was unaware that any of this was going on; I thought that I was just becoming sick again.

I had not yet learned that the body is often used as a tool for the old nature to justify its tenuous realities. That connection wasn't made yet. I still thought I was my body.

However, repressed righteous indignation, stronger than repressed anger (which is a counterfeit) was destroying my body and eating me up alive. I was weak from spiritual blindness. My denial of my true self was so overwhelming, I felt as if I were being pulled down by a powerful undertow at sea. I was watching myself drown. I did not have the power to stop it.

> Romans 7:18: "For I know that in me (that is, in my flesh)
> dwelleth no good thing: for to will is present with me;
> but how to perform that which is good I find not."

## Things Turned Around

At first I was the one taking care of "poor Tommy," until victimization, like a contagious virus, would make me the needy one. Soon I needed help from a friend, a therapist … a doctor. I had become totally disconnected from my new peaceful self. I had been taken out!

Tommy would stand by my side, loyal and noble, as I went straight down to the smallest me I could possibly be. Soon, he would be rescuing me!

> 1 Corinthians 10:14: "Wherefore, my
> dearly beloved, flee from idolatry."

## Doctor, I Lost My Kingdom!

I know that I am not alone here. I know that countless people have almost died here in this unidentified spot. Many who have come in for ministry have been through this exact set of circumstances. Most people do not express their problems from an accurate perspective.

As a minister and psychologist, I have never heard anyone blatantly declare, "I am suffering from a generational dysfunction!" Rarely (in the midst of an oppression) is a person able to ascertain with great insight and prophetic wisdom the truth of their situation. Few can acknowledge at that crucial point that they have been in a spiritual battle, stemming from a codependency, which later blossomed into idolatry. No one reports spiritual facts. If they did, it would sound something like this: "I was deceived into bowing to the past by a familiar spirit. After that, of course, I lost my Kingdom position and then was thrown back into the old creature's generational identification. My new seed, with all its power and opportunity, has been overcome."

No one describes his or her problems accurately. We are distracted by medical diagnoses. Spiritual problems are described as cancers, lupus, fibromyalgia or any number of illnesses. People will believe and confess, "I have arthritis. I have colitis. I have allergies, etc." Our health problems are not what they appear to be. They occur mostly in the unidentified spiritual warfare of codependency.

We are conditioned to disregard our relationships as being the cause of our health problems. We believe that our bodies get sick on their own as if they have lives separate from us — as if our interactions with each other as human beings are meaningless.

## Spiritual Misidentification

The number one killer in America is spiritual misidentification — most of it rooted in codependency. We give up our essence, our purpose, for the illusion of carnal love in exchange for the promise of emotional security and wholeness. This deception received gives the impostor a great opportunity to severely oppress our essence.

*Romans 7:15: "For that which I do I allow not: for what I would, that do I not; but what I hate, that do I."*

*Romans 7:17: "Now then it is no more I*
*that do it, but sin that dwelleth in me."*

Sin is in the old creature that lives in us all. It is our enemy, not our truth or identity. The spirit person always triumphs in liberty. Sometimes we just need to switch sides.

## My Spirit Was Prophetically Threatened

My spirit knew and was threatened even by Tommy's very presence. I would feel a physical shake or turmoil in my heart. All of me — my soul, my energy, my peace — would flee when he walked into a room. My spirit and God understood that as I engaged in this relationship, I would become so entangled in illusion and deception that I would lose my newfound perspective and understanding. I was initially standing separate from my past by grace. I had absolutely no conception that something else was going on besides Juliana and Tommy in a relationship.

After awhile, my eyes were no longer on my spiritual awakening.

*Romans 7:5: "For when we were in flesh,*
*the motions of sins, which were by the law, did*
*work in our members to bring forth fruit unto death."*

## I Had Problems

I had health problems. I had sleep problems. I had bowel problems. I was not moving ahead. I was being pulled back until finally there was no health. There were no bowel movements. There were no menstrual cycles. I was no longer ambulatory. All of my life forces had been totally oppressed.

I lost the healing and my recovery from the sauna detoxification program. I was toxic again. Only this time I would learn what toxicity truly was!

*Romans 7:11: "For sin, taking occasion by the*
*commandment, deceived me, and by it slew me."*

47

# Chapter 8

## My Definition of Toxicity

I had lost my spiritual connection and relinquished my grace! I knew nothing of spiritual forces manipulating through men and women to gain power over the soul. I knew nothing of holding onto or watching my power. I had no knowledge of generational beliefs.

## Generational Beliefs

Somewhere in my personal generational arsenal was an oppressive belief that my life had to be sacrificed for someone else's — that my life on its own could not freely be lived. I had to give up my life for a man, a friend or a parent. Another person would control my life. I was supposed to fulfill someone else's needs, take care of another person. My existence on its own merit had been rendered unimportant.

It was a spiritual battle. Generationally deceptive spirits with their beliefs of idolatry and condemnation had been handed down through the carnal bloodline from the carnal seed itself. It was passed from my mother and father, all the way back through generations of lifetimes. I am not talking about past lives of mine. I am talking about my ancestors' lives. I am talking about their level of truth, their spiritual development, their awareness and sanctification. These deceptions were derived from an inherited sin consciousness.

These same inherited deceptions would come back to challenge me as I emerged as my new self. They would try to take me back, pull me down and oppress my destiny. This was the war between the flesh and the spirit.

This law of guilt was the master of my flesh, my old nature. I was, however, the righteousness of God in Christ. We were not in agreement.

*Romans 8:3: "For what the law could not do, in that it was weak through the flesh, God sending his own Son in the likeness of sinful flesh, and for sin, condemned sin in the flesh."*

I would have to choose this day whom I would serve. I would have to pick one, to obey God or the idol. I would have to turn on this lie, tell it that I knew who I was, and confront it. But first I needed to understand my authority over it. The impostor would have to come under the subjection of my regenerated spirit. This was why God was telling me to stay free, detached, disentangled. I was not yet sanctified sufficiently for intimacy.

*Joshua 24:15: "Choose you this day whom ye will serve."*

## Call It Like It Is

In order to advance myself in my generationally inherited dilemma, I would have to see evil at the inception. Like a good baseball player, I needed to watch the ball and have my bat up, ready to clobber it. I would have to spiritualize my perceptions and learn to recognize deception by how I felt. None of this could be seen in the natural world, where it looked as if Tommy was perfect (most everyone agreed how lucky I was). Tommy was wonderful! He was always at my side willing to drive me to my abundance of doctors' appointments.

The rules had changed. Now that I was a spiritual contender, I had evil in the wings, waiting for me to fall. We were gambling for high stakes. One of us would take over, get the body and get the soul. One of us would survive. At the end of this battle, I would become a vessel for someone.

*Romans 6:14: "For sin shall not have dominion over
you, because ye are not under the law, but under grace."*

## The Love of God

Walking in love is a great spiritual concept. It is not so difficult to tap into the love of God. *"The Holy Ghost sheds the love
of God abroad in our hearts." (Romans 5:5)*

What is difficult is holding on to it. You cannot walk in the
love of God if you are unable to set boundaries and take care of
yourself. It is not possible to live in the grace of God with a
closed heart. If you do not set boundaries and take care of yourself, your heart will suffer for your ignorance.

*Proverbs 4:23: "Keep thy heart with all
diligence; for out of it are the issues of life."*

## Which Self Are You Taking Care Of?

To keep my heart in unconditional love, I would have to
know who I was. This meant being able to identify and choose
which self I was bringing into a relationship and making sure
that I was taking care of my spiritual self. To stay out of codependency, I would have to be very closely led by God and do
everything in God's timing. The agenda of man would have to
surrender to God's plan.

*Romans 6:9: "For ye are not in the flesh, but in the spirit,
if so be then that the spirit of God dwell within you."*

## Spiritual Power Attracts Light and Opposition:
## The Opposition Knows Your Battle

The opposition to your faith knows that moving ahead has
faith in it. This action of faith will empower you sufficiently to
bring the flesh under subjection. *Once you bring the flesh under
subjection, you have taken the law.* The law is powerless when

you are in your spiritual position of righteousness. Your spirit has dominion over sin consciousness (condemnation and guilt) and the curse of the law.

*Romans 8:1: "There is therefore now no condemnation to them which are in Christ Jesus, who walk not after the flesh, but after the Spirit."*

*Romans 8:2 "For the law of the spirit of life in Christ Jesus hath made me free from the law of sin and death."*

## You Can Miss the Mark

*If you felt you could make a mistake, that you could move in a wrong direction and still be blessed, you would not have fear.* If you believed that God would turn all things around for good, you would not have "fear of condemnation."

If every time you err you are to be punished, you will have tremendous fear of being misled. You will have an unconscious "fear of" walking out your door. It is a con of the impostor to undermine your identity and the grace of God simultaneously. The impostor will first attempt to maliciously mislead you, then blame and condemn you for the error it created! It will kick you when you are down and oppress you for learning how to be led!

*Romans 3:24: "Being justified freely by His grace through the redemption that is in Christ Jesus."*

## You Are Boss

The impostor's con of codependency opens every possible door for the old nature to rule. Furthermore, the slave of sin consciousness becomes your master! The old creature can begin to rule you, the spirit person.

You, here by divine appointment, summoned by a holy calling, taking nothing for or from yourself (your old self), you,

the righteousness of God in Christ, who have been given dominion over all things, who have been translated into His Perfect
Law of Liberty and saved by grace, can still become oppressed if
you do not enforce your grace and proper identity! It is possible
— even though you have every divine right on earth — to be
undermined, bullied, and intimidated into entering into bondage
as a slave. You may suddenly find yourself under the subjection
of, and doing the biddings of, evil. *This is not self-sabotage; this
is war. It is imperative to remember who is the boss at all times!*

> *Corinthians 15:45: "The first man Adam was made
> a living soul the last Adam a quickening spirit."*

## Impostor Inquisition

Another way to define codependency is as a belief in the
lack of the love of God. This belief is handed down from generations of sin consciousness. This fear of the lack of love of God
is an illusion created by the law. This adversary may then throw
in its mortal love, hoping you'll go for it. The impostor knows
that if it keeps you out of authentic connections long enough,
you might bite at this temptation.

Mortal love is not real. It is a counterfeit, like all carnal
attributes and qualities, and is a cheap impersonation of your
very real goods! This is why perfect love casts out fear and carnal love brings fear in. Carnal love adds to its disharmony the
utter disconnection from your Kingdom in God!

After several distractions, you might experience an intellectual mental idol attempting a conversation in your mind, having
you falsely concerned about its premeditated disconnection.

Pondering the what, why and how of this alleged disconnection gets one even further lost. These questions are the types of thoughts used in the "impostor inquisition." If these thoughts are received, they will create more fear, more disconnection. *Adding idols, after all, is deception's main theme.* You can be stuck up in your head trying to figure this whole thing out while the impostor is stealing your time. This is the impostor cleverly warring with you for your moment.

*1 Corinthians 2:11: "For what man knoweth the
things of man, save the spirit of man which is in him?"*

*1 Corinthians 2:14: "But the natural man receiveth not the
things of the spirit of God: for they are foolishness unto him:
neither can he know them for they are spiritually discerned."*

# Chapter 9

## An Inauthentic Fake

The carnal counterfeit nature, being an innate deception, has no genuine expression. It has no authenticity. It is faking and conning. Your power over it is to simply bust this con.

*1 Corinthians 1:29: "That no flesh should glory in his presence."*

## Busting the Inner Con

If the regenerated spirit person is to walk in consistent love, he or she must expose the con of the old nature! Once the con is identified, the spirit has automatic power over it. A spiritual person must call the con exactly what it is, thereby separating the con from one's true self!

If you do not call it and separate yourself from it, you can be manipulated into believing that you are the impostor. You could then be seduced into not upholding your righteousness!

*Romans 7:6: "But now we are delivered from the law,*
*that being dead wherein we were held; that we should*
*serve in the newness of spirit and not in the oldness of letter."*

## More on Carnal Love

Carnal love cannot be felt. It is not available in a tangible way. It might be released as physiological phenomena in the bedroom and is often mistaken for great passion and depth. Mortal love is not a fruit of the spirit — it has no authentic feelings. It is not capable of giving anything positive. How can it be?

Romans 8:5: *"For they that are in the flesh do mind the things of the flesh and they that are after the spirit the things of the spirit."*

## It Is Pretending to Be You!

The carnal nature is a fake. A bully. It is an impostor! Only authentic expression has the capacity to keep the heart open. Your heart responds to words.

We have all experienced hearing someone speak and suddenly feeling numb or dead because there was no feeling in the words. Our hearts automatically respond to a lack of authenticity in words. When someone begins to speak without feeling, without heart, the atmosphere soon goes dead. Words without "the ring of truth" are felt by everyone's heart. A person whose communication has not evolved to authenticity (an expression of their heart) is constantly shutting his or her own heart down.

Love cannot flow from a shutdown heart. There are, of course, levels of open and shut hearts. Train your ears to hear the spirit of words. Once you develop your spiritual hearing of thoughts and words, you will be able to bust the inner con and get a better sense of the lies and fears the impostor is using to attack your heart and spirit.

The ability to hear will keep you in God's moment. You will become more spiritually aware. Hearing is coming out of darkness and denial! There is a "fear of hearing" in the carnal nature; hearing is a threat. Take your true hearing back. Your hearing and expression of words represents who you are, your essence.

You cannot find someone whose expression you like and mimic it. You will not advance. You will have less authenticity and less heart. You will have more deception and self-justification.

Faith is the highest form of expression. The impostor is not excited about faking faith. It is a hard thing to fake!

This evil counterfeit is always warring against you for position, trying to make you forget that you have the love of God.

## The Impostor Hates You

The opposition to you and God knows that the illusion of carnal love is a big trap on this earth. It is actually hate! It is a tried and true setup to be conned and fall from grace. Hate, resentment, pain, and hurt are not fruits of love.

## Mental Idols

You are in mental codependency if another person is continuously in your thoughts and your mind is focused on them and their problems. Lay it down! Disengage from this person and change your plan. Fast!

No man or woman will ever survive the mental battle that codependency will bring without piggybacking onto the victory of Christ. You will be extinguished. When you have been deceived into a mental jam, you need grace! A mental jam is really an attack of the spirit of condemnation that attempts to create doubt and confusion in your purpose! It is a ploy of the generational arsenal of identification error to pull you back into who you are not.

> Romans 8:1: *"There is therefore now no condemnation to them which are in Christ Jesus ..."*

## Perceptions of Grace

Grace will look at an unsanctified person and not expect much from them. Grace understands that they are babies in the spirit and can accept them, love them and enjoy them just where they are.

The important thing is that you see the truth and are not conned by deceptions of the flesh.

You do not need to have long talks about working it all out with spirits of entanglement. You have nothing to work out. You are redeemed! If you are aware of this, you will not get entangled with them. You can live on this earth in the spirit of God, hid in Him. The answer will not be found in trying to work it out. A more Godly solution can more often be found in expansion, by moving on and getting out of the carnal agenda of codependency.

*Psalm 136:24: "And hath redeemed us from our enemies: ..."*

## The Big Impostor Guilt Trap (Victim Hook)

Do not get hooked into feeling the carnal emotions of grief, pity, sorrow or being sad. These feelings are a sure sign of being manipulated by sin consciousness. It is not your responsibility to rescue victims.

The voice of guilt will always have you focus on what another person wants and needs and what they are going through (as if you are undeserving of your rights). The voice of guilt will want you to stay in a situation when you want to go and will want you to go when you want to stay! It opposes you at all times by desiring always to create a mental conflict.

*1 Corinthians 9:11: "If we have sown unto you spiritual things, is it a great thing if we shall reap your carnal things?"*

## The Perceptions of Guilt

Just as the perceptions of grace are different, in a different dimension, so are the perceptions of evil. The dimension of deception is feigned, tainted and illusionary. The perceptions of guilt will seek to overcome your own perceptions and your true voice. Guilt will seek to silence all of your Kingdom power and connections. The law seeks to make you a sitting duck for perceptual error and then take the opportunity to lead you astray.

*2 Peter 3:17: "Ye therefore, beloved, seeing ye know these
things before, beware lest ye also, being led away with
the error of the wicked, fall from your own steadfastness."*

## Disagree with Guilt

Once you identify the voices of guilt and condemnation, you
have the authority to silence them. This begins by hearing the
voices, but not agreeing with them. Do not be silenced! Take a
stand and fight the good fight of faith.

*Ephesians 6:13: "Wherefore take unto you
the whole armour of God, that ye may be able to
withstand in the evil day, and having done all, to stand."*

## The Voice of Condemnation

The voice of condemnation is another enemy of you and
God. The voice of condemnation will undermine you in everything you do. It will speak insecurity to you, attempting to make
you less than who you truly are.

The spirits of self-justification and self-exaltation desire to
weaken your identity and steal your faith in God's plan for your
life. It is a faith battle. The carnal nature will utilize a subtle
inner verbal attack. It is that same arsenal of evil that the Lord
Jesus Christ has delivered you from. You do not have to tolerate
these deceptive undermines, feelings, hurts or misleadings. You
will, however, have to recognize them in order not to receive
them.

Your position is to identify and *not receive* the guilt and generational condemnation that wars within you. You have the
power to bust this con and arrest its attempt to oppress your
essence. This is also true with the carnal cons that may come
from the expressions and thoughts of people close to you.

## The Tables Turned

In my own situation, unidentified guilt and condemnation finally took their toll. I was being manipulated by the spirit of self-justification to forget who I was. My new self was submerged. Tommy eventually became much stronger and got on with his life, adjusted to his new environment and began developing businesses.

He was getting a life and I was losing one! I was becoming helpless and sick, getting more allergic to everything every day. I was learning a lot about toxicity. I just wasn't connecting with it yet. This was my environmental illness. I had been overtaken in the spiritual realm. I had gone completely unconscious!

My generational past had overcome my true nature. I had spiritually collapsed! I was out of my purpose. I could not keep the law out of my life. I had no resistance to generational guilt! I would have to learn to keep myself separate from condemnation and guilt to hold a healing. A healing is, after all, in grace. I was unknowingly bowing to evil. The law of sin and death reigned in my life for another season.

## Adding Idols

It was from this place that I went all the way down to total victimization and, finally, isolation.

I kept adding idol after idol. The old nature and its inherent self-exaltation took me on a journey of spiritual defeat. I became a seeker of doctors, dentists and many other illusionary treatments to get well. They were really just more attempts to treat who I was not.

*2 Corinthians 6:16: "And what agreement hath the temple of God with idols? For ye are the temple of the living God."*

59

## I Was Diagnosed

After seeing numerous doctors and holistic healers, I was diagnosed. It was apparent that I was allergic to everything. (They couldn't detect the psychic sensitivities — just the foods and chemicals.) Moreover, all the blood and allergy tests confirmed that I was a "universal reactor."

The amazing thing is that medical tests will agree with deception. They are just more validation, more justification for error. Where were the spiritual evaluations?

I had not yet received any of those lessons that day when I ordered my "last supper." I had not recovered from the deception of the law.

*Deuteronomy 11:16: "Take heed to yourselves,*
*that your heart be not deceived, and ye turn*
*aside, and serve other gods, and worship them."*

# Chapter 10

## The Food Arrived

I heard the delivery truck stop in front of my house. I rose from my seated position and quietly ran to hide in the bathroom. I was fearful of having any contact with the delivery person. I had a plan, a goal, and I wanted no complications. I tiptoed into the bathroom and silently shut the door. I would wait it out.

I heard the scotch tape being pulled off the envelope on the garage door. My delivery was made as instructed; all was going well. The driver walked back to his truck and left. I would wait until all the truck fumes had dissipated from my yard. When I felt the turf was clear, I ran out quickly, grabbed the bag, ran back into the house and slammed the door behind me.

## Food!

I had it in my hands! Food! I had ordered food! That reality distracted me momentarily from my concern about the possibility of truck-fume contamination.

## Unwrapping the Package

Carefully, with white cotton-gloved hands, I placed the forbidden food on my environmentally safe, old wooden snack table. I had already deposited my arsenal of drugs on that same table. Every item had been strategically placed so that I could eat and enjoy my "last supper" in peace. I had within my reach my lethal dose of drugs for the very instant I would have an allergic reaction. I could not take the risk of leaving the table in allergic shock. I would protect myself from receiving any additional pain. Then, suddenly, I was able to breathe more easily; I felt my lungs and chest relax.

## The Meal Itself

The meal I ordered was roasted chicken, French fries, onion rings, coleslaw and, for dessert, apple pie. I had nothing to lose if I were to eat and then die. I did not remove my gloves to eat. I still had to touch the bag and the aluminum foil in which everything was wrapped.

I picked the food out of its wrappings, holding small napkins cut in half. I didn't want to die with dirty gloves on. I was so hungry that I shook as I picked up my piece of roasted chicken. I ate wholeheartedly! I got so involved with eating that I almost lost sight of why I was able to partake in this feast.

## I Had My Feast

I would like to be able to report that I ate with style, with music, and with God. But the truth is, I did not enjoy every bite. I did not savor each moment. I did not laugh and cry. I simply gobbled it down, and then it was over.

## Waiting to Die

All I could do was wait. I have no idea why I didn't just take the pills after my meal was complete. I had no intention of being rescued. I had decided to eat and then, the minute the reaction hit, take all my pills and be unconscious in minutes, dead within an hour. It didn't matter how long it actually took to die. No one would find me. I would be in a passed-out position — no pain, no awareness. I would die from an overdose of barbiturates.

## More Waiting to Die

I had nothing to do but wait for the reaction. Usually, they were fairly immediate and long-lasting. I waited ... ten minutes passed, and I did not feel any inner shaking ... not yet. I did a physical inventory.

Was my stomach churning? Migraine? The usual. Nothing had worsened. Dizzy? Nausea? How were my muscles? Any spasms? Not yet ... I didn't feel good, but I was not any sicker than usual. Another ten minutes passed by, and I was still waiting for the more serious reactions.

My rationale for my delayed reaction was that my system hadn't eaten in so long that it would take longer to digest, to recognize food. Another fifteen minutes went by, a total of thirty-five minutes, and no reaction.

I was numb. One hour passed, and I still had no reaction to the enormous meal I had just eaten. I was so exhausted from the whole waiting-to-die routine that I decided to go to sleep.

I remember thinking, *If I live through the night* (which was very unlikely after such a huge meal — a meal that consisted of nothing but food to which I was violently allergic), *if by some rare possibility I am still alive in the morning, I will eat breakfast and then, when the reaction comes, I will kill myself.* I planned to eat very close to the snack table where I still had my entire stash of barbiturates. Tomorrow, I would eat and die.

## Eating and Dying

The next morning I found that I had survived the night none the worse for wear. I was alive, and I had eaten food! I was not that excited about being alive. I was still oppressed, lifeless.

Numb and disgusted, I intended to return to my original plan ... eat and die. Just because I had eaten and didn't die did not mean that I would be diverted from my path. I would not be so easily deterred. I was finished with my disempowered lifestyle. I would eat breakfast — and then die.

## Eat Breakfast and Die

I ate breakfast and didn't react! I ate lunch and didn't react! I decided that I would continue to eat until the reaction came, and then I would kill myself. I ordered more food. I ate dinner! I began to react, but mildly. I hadn't had this much water or food in so long that my body started to swell. I began to resemble the Elephant Man. My tiny legs started looking like huge tree stumps. My body was swollen and bloated. Nevertheless, I was eating, and I was alive. I had no explanation for this. I wanted to eat and die, and I was eating and living!

Unbeknownst to myself, I had taken a stand. It was clear that I had called a bluff. The mountain was moving. I prayed for understanding. I was expecting some kind of esoteric response. I didn't get it. It was as if God looked down from heaven to search the world for the most powerless person on earth, some-one with nothing: no food, no furniture, no clothes, no friends, no resources — a burnt-out broken vessel … He found me.

*Philippians 3:10: "That I may know him
and the power of his resurrection."*

## This Is Living?

Initially, just eating was satisfying enough. My original reason to end my life had gotten lost in the new agenda of eating. The change of plan from dying to eating and living had taken me totally by surprise. I no longer had a reason to end my life. I was no longer dying. I was living. I would be able to survive.

As time went on, I gained weight and my life was no longer threatened by a death of starvation. But, although I had been eating for a couple of months, I was beginning to become despondent again. I sat in my old, 100% wooden, nontoxic rocking chair, and began to think about my progress.

*Big deal,* I thought, *I am able to eat! But I am still too sensitive to leave my house, to be around other people. I am still a prisoner of my diseases.*

When I did eat, I would react. I was still feeling sick; the reactions were not severe enough to arrest my eating. I started to get discouraged again. I had never lived to eat and yet that was about all I was doing now.

At first, I was so grateful to be alive; it was enough. But now I longed to share with others, to connect, to express myself and be in the company of other human beings. I still could not tolerate any chemicals. The smallest chemical exposure would cripple me for days.

I was feeling very negative, hopeless and trapped. I was in solitary confinement, day in and day out — never a change, no visitors, no phone calls, no plans, no future. Perhaps I was just feeling sorry for myself ...

Then, in the midst of my pondering, a new thought interrupted my despair and I found myself thinking a thought I did not create, nor comprehend — a thought whose inception was from another consciousness.

The revelation I received that day was exactly this: *"My spirit's purpose in this life is to be in impeccable emotional and spiritual integrity simultaneously."* I had no idea what that meant. Frankly, I was not impressed. *So what?* I thought, *Impeccable what? I can't leave my house. How can I fulfill a purpose?* I simply discarded the thought and went to bed depressed.

# Chapter 11

## A Seed Was Released

When I awakened the next morning, I realized that it was not an eat-and-die day. Far from it ... this was a day of Glory! I noticed the difference the minute my eyes opened! I felt a peace. I stepped off my glass table bed with a new bounce! I was not inundated with negativity. I was looking forward to getting up, to facing my day. I was actually enthusiastic and energetic.

I was not used to having energy. Morning was my worst time; I woke up in isolation, with nothing to do but survive. I would prepare a meal, put a mask on to go outside and cook on my little electric hot plate, sit around and ponder my lot ... my activities were not inspirational.

There was something strange about my mornings. Usually I would awaken feeling as if I had been worked over during the night, as if I had been in a battle and lost. My body was always sore from the lack of a pillow, blanket and bedding.

This morning was different. I didn't recognize my energy or my thoughts. I had been changed in the night. I was a new person — renewed, resurrected, made over. This was the top-of-the-line me. I felt good. I had never felt this good before! Everything was different — my walk, my attitude, my faith, my hope, my mind. I wasn't getting the intimidating thoughts of fear. I didn't have my usual morning attack of terror.

I understand now that terror is a spiritual fear, the spirit knowing, screaming, "I'm not in my purpose, I am moving in a wrong direction! I am in danger!"

That morning I innately knew that I was moving in a right direction. Somehow, the right direction had found me! Who was I? Who was this? I was not my old self. I was somebody else. It felt like another being had come into my body and was living in me.

But it was me; it was not a feeling of possession. My will was in total agreement. I was new, fresh, very alive ... radically alive. I felt new life surging through me. This new life had a new power, a spiritual power. The power of God was apparently living in me and pouring through my veins, my heart, and lifting me above my own mind.

For the first time in a decade, I was excited about living! I had hope. What had created this change? Was it from a dream? A prayer? I had done nothing to facilitate this change. I had had no dreams, had seen and talked to no one, and still intervention had occurred!

## A Revelation on the Revelation

After contemplating all day, trying to "get" what had happened, the understanding flashed through my mind. I was given a revelation to explain the revelation. I realized that it was the word, the thought I had received the night before. That word was the reason for this new elevation! I had actually been born again in my own living room, sans prayer, sans church, and sans my own awareness.

I was born again, no doubt about it. A word, a thought, a revelation, had raised me from the dead — a word given to me in a moment of personal despair, in my own home, on a wooden rocking chair, in isolation.

*Romans 10:17: "So then faith cometh by*
*hearing, and hearing by the word of God."*

# Born Again

*1 Peter 1:23: "Being born again, not of corruptible seed,*
*but by the word of God, which liveth and abideth for ever."*

I tried to remember the strange word, something about my spirit's purpose and destiny. *That must be important,* I thought, *the spirit's purpose.* I recalled the word, *"My spirit's purpose is to be in impeccable emotional and spiritual integrity simultaneously."*

That was the key to my resurrection. I was born again by the revelation of my spiritual purpose.

I was translated from my human condition into the spirit person I was meant to be by the Word of God, spoken to my heart. God had released my destiny in the form of a revelation. The incredible thing that was my spirit had recognized it and awakened! My spirit knew that I had a chance now. I was renewed. I had a purpose. I was important to God. I had something to do, a destiny! I had backup. I was not alone anymore. I had God, helpers, maybe even an angel or two.

Yes, I had more than I had yesterday, that was for sure. God was interested in my life and me. Not only wasn't I dying, I had new life. I was born again, and now God Himself had taken a personal interest in my purpose! Things were looking up.

*1 Corinthians 15:22: "For as in Adam all die,*
*even so in Christ shall all be made alive."*

# The School of the Spirit

I was about to enter into the school of the spirit. I became a student of God, a very willing student. I focused of all my attention on my mission. I did not understand the revelation, this word that had divided my soul from my spirit and my mind from my fears. This word that had given me new life was incomprehensible to me.

*Hebrews 4:12: "For the word of God is quick, and powerful, and sharper than any two-edged sword, piercing even to the dividing asunder of soul and spirit, and of joints and marrow, and is a discerner of the thoughts and intents of the heart."*

I didn't understand it, but I liked it. I had no idea what God was talking about. I assumed that it was a "know as you go" system, and I waited to learn. I felt as if God were spending all of His time with me, instructing me, and I began to wonder if there wasn't anyone else out there that God needed to attend to! It was an amazingly intimate experience.

## My First Lesson (Spirit 101)

God wanted me to understand that I was insane. It seemed imperative to God that I realize that every thought I had was a deception and that everything I believed was a lie. I had no truth and no way to discern deception. This had a very humbling effect on me. I took this very personally. I was crazy! That was my problem! Diagnosed not by physicians or psychiatrists but by the maker Himself.

I had a false reality! I did not have lupus, food allergies, chemical sensitivities, or mercury toxicity. God wanted to be very clear here. I did not have any illness! I was, in fact, not my body! My body was an instrument that obeyed me. These illnesses were created by thoughts in my mind. My body was responding to thoughts and beliefs. I had been deceived.

## The Human Condition

I didn't realize at the time that God was revealing to me the intricacies of the carnal mind, and that every human being was in this madness. It was the condition of mankind. If I could see it, I could someday separate myself from it.

**69**

Right then, my little tiny baby step was to lay it all down. I was led to believe that I was insane. After seeing this, hearing this, admitting to this, I cried for six weeks! I took it hard. After the grieving period for my loss of sanity was over, I became motivated to surrender.

What had I to lose? God was willing to take my insanity for His Mind, no problem and no resistance. I was totally broken down. I was humbled. I was grateful, in fact, for the opportunity to lay my illusions down.

*Ephesians 4:23: "And be renewed in the spirit of your mind."*

## Surrender the Old Nature

I surrendered every deception I had to God, thought by thought.

*2 Corinthians 10:5: "Bringing into captivity every thought to the obedience of Christ."*

## Holiness

I came to understand who I really was, and that I was not crazy at all. God was teaching me how to separate myself from the thoughts and deceptions of the carnal mind, from the human condition and beliefs of the world. I was ready to stand in my new position as the righteousness of God in Christ. I was ready for some lessons. I was predestined to mature in faith.

# Chapter 12

## Spiritual Battles

I was finding that, in the spiritual realm, all serious contenders know exactly what is going on. A victim of an oncoming spiritual attack is the last to know! Once your regenerated spirit gets a sense of its power, you are no longer a victim — you are quite naturally a warrior. That's what Jesus means when He refers to us as the army of God: trained soldiers, able to *identify evil and retaliate.*

*Ephesians 6:10-12: "Finally, my brethren, be strong in the Lord, and in the power of his might. Put on the whole armour of God, that ye may be able to stand against the wiles of the devil. For we wrestle not against flesh and blood, but against principalities, against powers, against the rules of the darkness of this world, against spiritual wickedness in high places."*

The fulfillment of destiny doesn't happen overnight. But you could not have convinced me of that in my new moment. I was feeling good again! I had every confidence that my consecration and surrender to the Holy Spirit would create absolute healing. I knew beyond any shadow of a doubt that God was walking me out of my diseases. He was with me, on my side. Here I was, alive. That could not be disputed.

*Philippians 1:21: "For me to live is Christ, and to die is gain."*

With the kind of radical aliveness I was experiencing, why would I suspect any foul play? Who was I to get paranoid with destiny, with purpose? In my small sphere of reality I knew this much: I was alive and I was getting out of my house! I was walking near chemicals and fumes that were previously intolerable. I was able to do this by bringing every thought to the obedience of Christ.

> *2 Corinthians 10:5: "Casting down imaginations, and every high thing that exalteth itself against the knowledge of God, and bringing into captivity every thought to the obedience of Christ."*

I was surrendering my entire carnal mind to God. Moment by moment, thought by thought, I would watch my thoughts and give them to God. Not an isolated fifteen-minute meditation, but all day long, every waking hour!

> *Luke 12:25: "And which of you with taking thought can add to his stature one cubit?"*

This was a time when I was finally out of my house and able to go into the marketplace and shop in stores again. One day, when I was out basking in my new freedom, I walked into a shop and saw and smelled fresh paint on the walls. My carnal mind made intimidating suggestions. *Look, look, over there. Oh my God, oh my God. Look, there's fresh paint on the walls! You react violently to that. You're going to get sick; you're going to get really sick. Get out. Get out! You'll be sick for days!*

I felt my body start to react, and I was led to intercede with thought and prayer, lifting my thought, my entire mind, to my Father in Heaven.

I watched and prayed, *My Father, this is not your will, and I surrender these lies of thought to you. I deny, My Father, the lies of my mind.*

That's all I had, that's all I knew! It was good enough! When I did this, my physical reactions dissolved. I was starting to make the spirit mind connection and see the power of the Spirit over the mind and over the body. *My spirit mind, my true mind, had dominion over my carnal human mind and over my physical body.*

*Ephesians 1:21: "Far above all principality, and power, and might, and dominion, and every name that is named, not only in this world, but also in that which is to come."*

## Surrender Brought Peace

This was a very joyful time — just to be outside, to walk among people, to go to a department store, to touch fabrics and to be able to eat food in restaurants. I was being raised from the dead, and I was very grateful. I knew I had a long way to go. I still wasn't able to buy normal clothes or move from an environmentally safe house. However, I was blossoming daily! Everything was new!

I had my surrender to God, and I was walking in grace. Every day brought me more strength, and I saw no reason for this process to change or end. I had the victory. I had surrendered to God. I was connected and hooked up to the Great I Am. I was free. God Himself was interested in developing my faith.

*Philippians 4:7: "And the peace of God, which passeth all understanding, shall keep your hearts and minds through Christ Jesus."*

## Refined by Fire

There were two ways to be refined by fire, I was quickly learning. One way was to wait to get attacked, distracted, blame circumstance (lose spiritual consciousness) and return to the insane denial system of the carnal mind. With that passive choice, I could easily be seduced by the spirit of self-justification to once again believe that I was suffering from things "outside" of myself: illnesses, devils, God, life, parents and past situations — all contrived deceptions.

*Romans 13:1: "Let every soul be subject unto the higher powers. For there is no power but of God: the powers that be are ordained of God."*

## Spirit Is a Volunteer Worker in Christ
## (A Natural Retaliator)

The more excellent way in my situation was to take a spiritual perspective: to acknowledge that I needed power; to acquiesce to God's plan and be grateful for it; to agree with God's opportunity; and, most importantly, to volunteer to create it. *I could choose to go into the fire. I could see the fire for what it was: a way to get spiritual authority.*

> *1 Corinthians 3:13: "Every man's work shall be made manifest: for the day shall declare it, because it shall be revealed by fire; and the fire shall try every man's work of what sort it is."*

I was dead and now alive by fire. I had more power via fire. This was God's resurrection plan for me, stepping out into the fire by faith. I wanted to fight the good fight of faith when I was attacked. I would not give up any healing ever again! I was excited about my new way of life. I desired to live my soul's purpose and grow in my divine seed. I would give my generational inherited identity a battle for its troubles. My Lord would empower me to become the new seed and live a new life with my regenerated spirit woman in her destiny.

> *Romans 4:13: "For the promise, that he should be the heir of the world, was not to Abraham, or to his seed, through the law, but through the righteousness of faith."*

I would not let evil steal any more of my life. As a matter of fact, I would counterattack by taking back my rightful dominion and retaliate for my trouble tenfold.

I would undo how I got sick.

## How I Got Sick (What Illness Is)

I had allowed my dominion and power to be diminished by beliefs of my physicality and erroneous identification of my spiritual nature. This was perpetrated by professionals who could not help me remember who I was. Medical and spiritual practitioners would willingly and unknowingly agree with my victimization here on earth.

The carnal nature took full advantage of my ignorance. It seized this opportunity to keep me out of my purpose for as long as it could. It chose a long and resourceful medical route to justify its lying symptoms. Much of it, I eventually realized, were idols of generational self-exaltation to further blind and oppress me.

We are all spirits. So, to be healed, we must be healed in who we are. We must be awakened to the inner battle. Sometimes the old nature has to hit bottom to submit. Often, the old nature will do a complicated avoidance, a running away from God. Finally, there is nothing left to try, and no fruit has been borne.

*Hebrews 7:16: "Who is made, not after the law of a carnal commandment, but after the power of an endless life."*

## Integrity Is Health

I came to understand that physical health and immune system function represent the barometer of integrity and righteousness in the human spirit! I found that when I was high on the barometer of condemnation and victimization, I was low on energy. When my barometer of integrity was high, I had tremendous aliveness and health. I was learning to watch these characteristics and to see their effect on my health. It was about taking care of my spiritual self.

*Psalm 26:1: "Judge me, O Lord; for I have walked in mine integrity: I have trusted also in the Lord; therefore I shall not slide."*

## The Old Nature Hangs On

Often in healing there is a give and take — a step forward, a victory, and then a counterattack. Today I understand this, and when I stand with a brother or sister who is retaliating, we are prepared. We have warfare strategies.

My situation was different. I was alone, and I had very little of God's Word (truth to war with) and no stand. I had tremendous challenges, resistances of the old nature. I had given up so much; my flesh was not going to relinquish its hold that easily. I had been generationally conditioned to victimization, and now I was being challenged to become the master of my own temple.

*2 Corinthians 6:16: "And what agreement
hath the temple of God with idols?"*

# Chapter 13

## Some Trials and Tribulations

Mastery (dominion) is not immediate. There was a time, one of many, when I became disconnected. I was unable to hear God's voice to be led. I understood that I was being healed by surrendering to God. I knew I was in grace, but when something happened, I didn't know how to receive God's grace or forgiveness. I didn't know how to stay sanctified (separate from my old nature). I would then get oppressed and feel confused. I didn't understand that this was simply an attack of the law via condemnation and guilt.

I was paying a price for error that had been paid for at the Cross of Calvary and had nothing to do with my personal behavior. It didn't matter whether I was good, bad, a nice person, right or wrong. I still believed that my actions, my righteousness or lack of it, could contribute to or take away from my grace and healing! I spent a lot of time diligently watching and trying to correct my behavior. The thief of my spiritual identity, the impostor of my being, was inherently grace-resistant.

*Ephesians 2:8: "For by grace are ye saved through faith; and that not of yourselves: it is the gift of God."*

## Resisting Grace

During one of these grace-resistant moments, I stepped outside the back door of my house and walked right into the spray from an insecticide-spewing hose that my neighbors had set up to protect their lawn from ants and other bugs. Our houses were close enough (for an environmentally sensitive person) that with a little downhill wind, I could taste the spray!

I have noticed that when grace is resistant, the curse takes the immediate opportunity to create misfortune. This is not God punishing us for being misled; *this is evil itself taking advantage of a soul in the school of the spirit*! In God's training program, there is only grace for grace. To grow in grace is an uphill continuum.

> *Hebrews 12:28: "Wherefore we receiving a*
> *Kingdom that cannot be moved, let us have grace."*

## Grace Resistance Can Be Overcome

When we are experiencing "grace resistance," we are simply oppressed and in an identity attack. We have been oppressed by being misled, weakened to receive error. We need "word restoration," or word replacement with love. Your heart needs to hear words of proper identification to return to the now. It is grounded in words, and it needs empowering words to feed its new life. Your spiritual translation (which is complete) is upheld by proper identification via *words and purpose*! You have to be reminded daily of who you really are and of the power of your Kingdom in Christ.

> *Colossians 1:13: "Who hath delivered us from the power of*
> *darkness, and hath translated us into the Kingdom of his dear son."*

## Don't Take My Word for It

God runs His universe on words! Words are an output of energies that come either from truth of the spirit or from generational deceptions. These are words you receive and allow to enter your thoughts. The words you choose to think, speak, hear and agree with are what you are creating in any moment. Words, or undermining thoughts, negate your true identity and attempt to steal your grace! Words of condemnation are the lowest form of thoughts and ideas on the planet. Words of guilt and victimization are in agreement with the law of sin and death!

These sin consciousness words are spoken into the atmosphere and into your heart. Repeating victimizations (verbally telling your story) over and over sends these words and their energies with their corresponding emotions back into your heart! It will not behoove you to express a victimizing tale from the viewpoint and mentality of victimization.

It is a plot of the law of sin consciousness itself to procreate, prosper, and survive in your life. Evil's goal is to literally take you down with negative words from your own mouth. Evil would like to use you and your words to proliferate its existence. Tell your story from who you are, your spiritual perspective, and if necessary, demonstrate your spiritual authority.

*Proverbs 6:2: "Thou art snared with the swords of thy mouth, thou art taken with the words of thy mouth."*

## Words of Fear and Doubt

In this new situation, my carnal mind panicked. There had been so many words spoken and received about the dangers of pesticide exposure. Pesticide exposure is, after all, considered by most toxicologists to be a chemical immune system disaster. Many people who have been exposed to pesticides never recover.

This awareness gave the impostor an opportunity to set me up with anxiety, doubt and panic. Evil wanted assurance of an identification turnaround; it wanted its position back as master. I listened to some very hostile threats and started getting sensitive to everything again.

If you have ever had the experience of bringing your carnal mind under subjection for a season you will understand exactly what I am talking about! I thought it was over. I honestly believed that I was dead in Christ.

If you have not had this experience, I will explain the nightmare that occurred as best I can. I lost my connection, my enlightenment, my identity, my separation, and my sanity.

> *Mark 1:13: "And he was there in the*
> *wilderness forty days, tempted of Satan …"*

## The Carnal Mind Attacked with a Vengeance

I could not stop my thoughts! My healing was about peace, grace and surrender. It was about letting go of all thoughts, concerns and burdens. It was so easy, so freeing. I had a wonderful connection to my Heavenly Father and to the Holy Spirit. All I had to do was let go and give it all to God … but I found that I couldn't let go!

I could not stop the torment that had literally taken over my mind! I had been overcome by panic. I had never experienced anything like this level of anxiety before: pure, unadulterated fear! I had never seen or heard my carnal mind provoked in this way. My thoughts sped up. I was used to my time being slowed down in Christ, and now my time was accelerated in the law. I was attacked at a level far above my understanding.

I had lost my surrender to God! I did not know how to get it back. There is something truly unraveling about having to go through something twice! I had been totally confident in God's plan; I thought I was healed. The Mind of Christ was in peace. This trauma, this stress, had activated and stimulated the return of my carnal mind. I went into utter chaos! I was overwhelmed!

> *Romans 8:6: "For to be carnally minded is death;*
> *but to be spiritually minded is life and peace."*

I could not comprehend what was happening. Before this attack, I had not one doubt that I was going all the way with God! I had been blessed and healed. I had done nothing to appropriate my gift and suddenly I was losing it. I went insane!

During my entire illness, depressed and deathly ill, I never had that kind of panic. It was demonic and unstoppable.

*Hebrews 4:16: "Let us therefore come boldly unto the throne of grace, that we may obtain mercy, and find grace to help in time of need."*

## I Began to Lose My Healing

All I could think was *I cannot go through this again. I don't have it in me. I cannot live like this again! I can't get sick again! I won't survive.*

My only other thoughts were obsessive. This is what my carnal mind sounded like every waking moment: *Where's God? Where is my God? Where is God! How could this happen? I have lost my surrender to God!*

I was unable to hear or receive anything. I was utterly disconnected from myself. I was tossed out of my own body. I had no ground without God! My total and only focus was on my lack of connection to God.

I was a woman without spiritual authority, fallen from grace. Spirits of doubt intimidated me without letup. I felt as if the plug that I needed to survive had been pulled. I wanted desperately to reconnect with God, to feel His Presence. I needed to be reconnected to the Holy Spirit. That would be the only thing that would satisfy me.

*Hebrews 3:8: "Harden not your hearts, as in the provocation, in the day of temptation in the wilderness ... "*

# Where Are You, God?

I did a "tour" of seeking help. I would attempt to explain my situation to pastors, ministers, and spiritual practitioners, somehow expecting everybody to understand my strange plight! I would look at them and cry out, "I've lost my surrender to God!"

I must have sounded like John the Baptist crying out in the wilderness: "Where is God?"

"Where did my surrender go? I have lost my surrender to God. How do you get it back?"

No one was relating to me. I was speaking such basic truth that I was frightening people, communicating on such a primal level. Perhaps I was identifying everyone's problem. I assumed that everyone had surrendered and was consecrated to a relationship with God. This assumption was bizarre in itself, albeit very real for me at the time.

In retrospect, I realized that I was speaking to people who probably hadn't surrendered to God. They did not have the ability to comprehend losing their surrender, much less advise me on retrieving mine. They could not understand my trauma; I was speaking a different language. They contributed many suggestions, such as: feel your feelings, forgive everyone, breathe more fully. None of it made sense to me.

The law was trying to seduce me further by interjecting the next level of temptation! It was trying to get me into some kind of process. "It's not about any of that," I would attempt to explain. "I had God. I walked in His grace via surrender and now I have lost my position, my God, my lifeline, my surrender to God."

Was that so hard to understand? It was. His grace had escaped me. I was lost again.

Every day, I was getting sicker, relinquishing more foods, getting chemical reactions again, losing all that I had gained. This went on for three months.

*2 Corinthians 4:11: "For we which live are always delivered unto death for Jesus' sake, that the life of Jesus may be manifested in our mortal flesh."*

# Chapter 14

## One More Time without Feeling

I experienced three long months of trying to surrender. I felt I had already surrendered everything. Surrender was my way to get to God, and surrender wasn't working. How could this be? These unanswered questions were impossible to purge from my mind. After all, the carnal mind would constantly remind me over and over, *You are not connected to God. Where is God?*

I felt as if I were starting to die again. This time things were different. I had tasted Glory, and I didn't want to die. I was not in agreement with the spirit of death. I wanted to find God and be led by His spirit and be in His grace once again. I knew then that all would be well.

*Romans 8:2: "For the law of the Spirit of life in Christ Jesus hath made me free from the law of sin and death."*

## I Have One Thing Left to Surrender

I remember sitting in a chair pondering my lack of surrender. I finally concluded that I would have to surrender trying to surrender! If surrender was my way to God, then that would be my last sacrifice! That was all that remained to be surrendered—surrender itself! I would give up even this last struggle.

*Hebrews 11:35: "Cast not away your confidence, which hath great recompense of reward."*

## I Surrender Surrendering

I started to observe from a new perspective: I would not surrender! I had my thoughts. I had my feelings. I had the desire to surrender. I began watching with this new awareness. I observed my thoughts. I chose to not surrender!

I started breathing a little more deeply. I repeated my new watch once more … What did I have left? I had my thoughts. I had my breath. I had my feelings. I had a desire to surrender. And I would not surrender. I would surrender the surrendering! I began to notice something else.

> *Hebrews 11:36: "For ye have need of patience, that after you have done the will of God, you might receive the promise."*

> *Hebrews 11:37: "For after a little while, and he that shall come will come, and not tarry."*

## My Thoughts Are Creating My Feelings!

By not surrendering my thoughts as I normally would, I noticed that my thoughts were creating my feelings. I had not been able to notice this when I was focused on my surrender agenda! I was being led again! The Holy Spirit was separating me so that I could observe a new thing, the next thing to learn.

As I chose to not surrender and continued to watch my thoughts, it was clear. It was fact — my thoughts were changing and controlling my feelings! My thoughts were controlling even my very breath!

I began having an epiphany. I continued to not surrender. As I surrendered trying to surrender, the more I was able to see what was really going on.

My thoughts were definitely creating my feelings. My feelings were reduced to mere symptoms of my thoughts! I was making an important connection, one that would change my life! I was in a move of God! I was inspired.

I continued. I watched. I had my thoughts. I had my breath. I had my feelings (responses from the latest thought). The feelings changed with the change of thought! I had been tormented by thought! I would not, however, surrender this thought! I would not surrender any emotions.

I began to have another round of feelings. This time there was a soul terror — a deeper, more primal terror.

The enemy of God was taking its last shot, creating an intense disharmony within, using some "throw me off course" feelings, trying to keep me from moving ahead. It was a last attempt to block me from retrieving my Kingdom.

I was holding on. Standing fast.

> Galatians 5:1: "Stand fast therefore in the
> liberty wherewith Christ hath made us free, and
> be not entangled again with the yoke of bondage."

I knew that I was going somewhere. I was being led to something. I could sense it in the spirit. The Holy Spirit directed me: *"Just say no. Just say no! Just say no to all your thoughts!"*

## Just Say No!

I had been spending every waking hour for three months trying to surrender— to yield all my feelings, all my thoughts, thought by thought, a process that God Himself had taught me. It was clearly over. I had been promoted! What was this "Just say no"? I was not certain.

I was, however, elated that I had finally heard something. God was talking to me again. *"Just say no! Just say no to the thought."* No. That's all, easy, just a big 'no.' Two letters and the panic was over. "No!"

I realized that I was being stressed out and brought down by emotions. By not receiving the preceding negative thought, I could arrest the entire negative emotional realm. Hallelujah!

The Lord instructed me further: "*I want you to die to all these victimizing thoughts. Split your mind up in two categories, power thoughts and victim thoughts; victim thoughts get a no. Any time an undermining or fearful thought about anything comes up, just say no. Just say no to undermining evil!*"

I had been given the weapon I needed. I didn't realize until I started saying "no" how often my mind was negative, undermining, and condemning. I became aware of the emotional pain and grief that that type of thinking created!

## I Say No a Lot

I negated every thought. I was vigilant. I had no choice. Within four days, I was out of the anxiety and all of the emotional pain and burdens that I had been living in. I became sane again. I felt as if a boulder had been lifted off of my soul. My energy returned, and my health decline was arrested.

I was out of the wilderness again, and I clearly saw the importance of always being willing to let go of something, anything that would take my peace, even for a moment. Nothing and no one was worth losing my moment. Letting go was faith and peace. The holding on had been the flesh plotting to take me back to its bondage.

I saw that my safety lay in the sacred moment of God, led by God, designed by God. Grace could only happen in God's plan. Grace could not be provoked or faked. Grace was the will and free gift of God!

The curse of the "law" is an irrevocably hostile instructor — every error was severely punished by a loss of health, peace, and the wasting of precious time. To learn from the law was a lesson itself in the need for grace.

*Galatians 3:23: "But before faith came, we were kept under the law, shut up unto the faith which should afterwards be revealed."*

*Galatians 3:24: "Wherefore the law was our schoolmaster to bring us unto Christ, that we might be justified by faith."*

# Enforcing Grace

I would not have relinquished my healing if I had enforced my God-given grace. The grace of God will hold you up! That grace is appropriated by faith. *"For by grace are ye saved through faith."* (Ephesians 2:8) The law of grace (The Perfect Law of Liberty) has all power over the law of sin and death.

I still had dominion on this earth, even though lying symptoms and opposing thought were influencing me. I could have demonstrated my authority over my body by confronting the pesticide. I since have done just that; I have actually slept in rooms that had just been sprayed with pesticides and, of course, the carnal nature bowed to my superior spiritual position!

*Battling to enforce grace is always the fastest way to come back into the spirit of God!* A little retaliation, upping the ante on the alleged problem, no matter what it is, automatically brings the victory that God has already purchased for us! How could it not? In only one way. I did not yet know about it.

*Galatians 3:29: "And if ye be Christ's, then are ye Abraham's seed, and heirs according to the promise."*

## Led by the Spirit

I had begun to get it. I was safe when God was leading; being led was a position of grace. Being led would cover what I couldn't see, didn't yet know. Being led would bring all of my ignorance under subjection; being led gave me the power of who I was becoming by grace. Being led made the future me, the me of spiritual regeneration, the now me. *"By the washing of regeneration, and renewing of the Holy Ghost." (Titus 3:5)*

It was like borrowing knowledge, power, wisdom and experience. It connected me with my true identity. I could be spared from repetitive learning and error by one immutable fact: *"But if ye be led of the Spirit, ye are not under the law." (Galatians 5:18)*

I would no longer allow any disturbance of my peace. The law had just tried to kill me again, but this time I was able to resist. I had refused temptation with one powerful God-given word. No.

*Matthew 5:37: "But let your communication be Yea, yea; Nay, nay: for whatsoever is more than these cometh of evil."*

**89**

# Chapter 15

## The Real Battle

The battle for the moment is very high and, ultimately, the only real battle you will ever need to know! If you can stay in the moment, you can be led. You are then in the Perfect Law of Liberty, and you will be upheld and blessed.

The moment battle is not clinging to a belief, or even fixing yourself. It is simply appropriating the moment by faith. A primal but very refined battle. How we do it changes more often than the carnal mind can imagine, and that's the point.

The carnal mind can never control it. The moment is sans agenda. The moment abides in liberty! The moment is God's Holy ground. It is your vehicle to walk out of denial and into the light via faith in God. In the sacred moment, there is no avoidance of what is really going on. There is no looking back, no past, no planning for the future. There is just you, your spirit, your mind, your choices, and God-given authority over your expression of truth. Your surrender to the moment holds for you the power of "The Cross of Christ," and your death and resurrection therein.

*Acts 7:33: "For the place where thou standeth is holy ground."*

## A Baby Step for Spirit Kind

I had taken authority over my surrender, my first move in stepping out more maturely in God. I now knew that surrender was not enough! I had gotten clobbered surrendering! I was unable to stay in His presence with just surrender! It was not enough of a weapon to surrender my thoughts only! How was that possible? Wasn't surrender my goal with God? Whatever the Holy Spirit was teaching me, I needed to learn.

## The Law Distracts Me Further

I had to move on. I had to get bigger than these attacks and setbacks. I knew that I had to take my will back in full faith and move on. I had missed the mark (the leading of the spirit), and that error, without the full understanding of God's grace, had opened the door to attacks. I had to learn how to not be tossed if I were to hold my healing and stay in the spirit.

*Ephesians 4:14-15: "Be no more children, tossed to and fro,*
*carried about with every wind of doctrine, by the sleight of*
*men, and cunning craftiness, whereby they lie in wait to deceive,*
*but speaking the truth in love, may grow up into him in all things."*

It was time to focus on moving ahead. I was not living as a healed person. I was still unable to move from my house to a normal residence. Normal meant a place with new carpet, fresh paint, house cleaning products, carpet shampoo — all the usual toxic chemicals of everyday life.

## The Flesh Takes Control

I did a final runaround, an avoidance of God's plan. Not conscious avoidance. Avoidance is not conscious. I bought into the impostor's concepts of dry, fresh air being the healer. I made the environmentally safe move to clean air in the high desert. Many chemically sensitive people had experienced some improvement by sleeping outside in dry, clean air.

I did one more final take of the safe housing and clean air illusion. None of it worked for me. It turned into hell. Wrong place, wrong time, no faith, and no grace. No new moment! Just the same old attempted carnal ways of trying to "fix" an illness, complying with beliefs about air quality, distracted into the fruitless battle of self. All vanity ... I was headed in a wrong seed direction — wrong identity, no blessings, no miracles, no healings. Let's face it: No faith!

> *Ecclesiastes 1:14: "I have seen all the works that are done under the sun; and, behold, all is vanity and vexation of spirit."*

## Hell Breaks Loose

I think we all know about doors opening being God, and doors closing not being a good sign. I would consider a fire breaking out in the forest directly across the street from the house where I lived a salient and potent sign of a door closing. The entire area was closed off and evacuated. Needless to say, the smoke did not help my plight.

> *Hebrews 11:38: "For the just shall live by faith: but if any man draw back my soul shall have no pleasure in him ..."*

## You Have Nothing to Lose

I returned to my nontoxic house in Santa Barbara. I was totally desperate again. I called Cynthia, an acquaintance who had once had environmental illness and had been healed. I thought she might know something. She had survived this nightmare and had taken her life back.

Cynthia suggested that I go to a service and meet a minister with whom she'd had a lot of healing. I had become so sensitive from the smoke in the desert that I couldn't even drive my car without wearing several masks.

To attend this meeting, I would have to drive from Santa Barbara to Westwood, California. "Cynthia, I can't do this drive! I don't have the strength for it," I told her. "The fumes alone will set me back for months. I don't know what to do. I can't eat. I haven't eaten in days. I can't get there! I am too sensitive! I'm stuck in my house!"

Cynthia replied, "Juliana, you have no choice. You have nothing to lose. Just get in your car and come here."

She reached me with that comment. She was absolutely right. She said the one thing that I had to agree with. Cynthia didn't try to talk me into anything, or tell me how great the minister was; she used the hard, cold fact that I had absolutely nothing to lose! Amen to that! I threw on my rags, wore three facemasks, and put the air conditioner on "high" to block incoming fumes.

I ventured to Westwood.

## Surrounded by Psychos

The meeting was held in the minister's home. The place was packed. People were lined up outside his door. All the rooms were full of people awaiting prayer.

Cynthia came out to the driveway to meet me and grabbed my arm to walk me inside. I could not enter the home! There was so much deodorant, perfume, dry-cleaning fluids — all chemicals that I still could not tolerate.

I was traumatized and ran back into the car. After over a hundred people had been prayed for, the minister came out. Many of the people had left. Pastor Tim and Cynthia got me out of my car again, and took me to an isolated area in a small room where I could be prayed for. I was surrounded by roughly twenty people (the "in crowd"); the inner circle was still present.

I couldn't recognize the different languages they were speaking. "How can they communicate with each other if they are not speaking the same language?" I thought. These people did not connect at all! I looked around, and suddenly I knew what it was; they were speaking in tongues! These were tongue talkers! They were babbling fast and in all kinds of different tongues.

I remembered seeing it on TV. I had no idea what they were talking about. At one point, Pastor Tim did an interpretation of one of the tongue languages they were speaking.

*I'll never get out of here alive*, I thought. *How is this going to help me?*

I was reacting violently to the perfumes, the deodorants, the hair spray, the people; I was crying desperately, screaming in utter torment. I looked up and thought, *This is the lowest place I've ever been in my life. I'm surrounded by psychos, and I'm hoping they're going to help me! I'm seeking help from mentally ill people!*

The minister was busy casting out my devils. I remember thinking, *How can I have gotten this low in my life? How? I am dying. I am so ill I cannot eat, and psychos are casting out devils.*

My devil belief was limited. I just wanted to die. *I would rather die than be this down, this lowly, this totally insane,* I thought. *I cannot do this. I cannot fake this. I cannot be a part of such insanity. I cannot compromise my heart, my soul, my integrity—all that is within me—to this level of psychosis. I am still a doctor, a psychologist; I know and am able to diagnose insanity when I see it, and I am seeing it! I am surrounded by it!*

My carnal mind did not like this crowd at all!

## Commanding Devils?

Pastor Tim stood right over me. I was on the floor, writhing, screaming in protest, freaked out!

"I command the spirit of death to go from her," Pastor declared. "By the blood of Jesus, come out. I command the spirit of infirmity to come out, come out! Come out now!"

He was screaming. Everybody was screaming something at this point! The helpers were all singing "The Blood of Jesus" loudly. Some were yelling it, some were making up some kind of melody and singing it, some were praying it.

Pastor Tim continued. "I command the spirit of fear to go. I command the spirit of torment to go from her. Come out, devil; come out, by the blood and the Holy name of Jesus!"

The background chants got louder, and they were all praying in tongues now. It sounded as if they were all hysterical, like a scene from *One Flew Over the Cuckoo's Nest*!

"By the Blood," they were screaming, "by the Blood of Jesus! The Blood of Jesus!"

Over and over, chanting, screaming, singing... *Is this devil deaf?* I wondered. I just wanted to go home and be sick and die in peace. I wanted out of this horrifying nightmare.

## I Am Mindless

Finally, the exorcism drama was over, and I wobbled back to my vehicle, spaced out. I practically fell into my car. I was having trouble thinking straight. I was totally unable to focus my mind.

At first, I felt that I was weakened by the insanity, by the scene itself. Perhaps my mind had just stressed out and shut down. Then I noticed: I had no thoughts! No thoughts at all! Could my thoughts have been removed? Exorcised?

My mind had been stopped, reprogrammed, its subject matter removed. My mind was blank!

I could not hear a thought. I was attempting to think, but my mind was not receiving my thoughts. It seemed as if my own thoughts were no longer available to my mind. I was still too stunned to consider what had just happened at Pastor Tim's house.

I couldn't! I had no comments, no opinions, no judgments. I could not form a thought!

## It's about Faith

Suddenly, in the car on the way home, I was overwhelmed by a repetitive thought. My mind felt as if it had been taken over, pushed aside by a greater force. Over and over again, like a broken record, I heard one thought and one thought only. My mind was repeating one solitary thought: *It's about faith,* my mind declared. *It's about faith.*

No matter how hard I tried, I could not think another thought! I was not choosing to think this. No other thoughts would come.

All the anxiety, fear and panic, all the trauma, all the disgust — gone! Nothing was left, no emotions involved, no terror. All I could hear was one thought, over and over. One thought repeating itself. *It's about faith.*

## I Eat by Faith

My carnal mind had been stopped, and the Spirit was now controlling it. There was a concept God Himself wanted me to grasp, a simple one: *"It's about faith."*

I found myself driving to the Melting Pot, a restaurant in Westwood, not far from the Pastor's home. I hadn't eaten in days, not a morsel! I got out of my car, and as if I did this every day, I walked in and ordered a normal meal. *After all,* I remember reasoning, *It is about faith!*

If it's about faith, it's not about food; it has nothing to do with food. If it's about faith, if I were hungry, I might as well eat, I somehow concluded. My one magnified thought continued to pervade my consciousness! I made a decision. *I will eat by faith!*

I ordered food and ate my first meal! I didn't think about it— I couldn't. I can't even remember what I ordered. It didn't matter. I actually digested the meal and drove home in peace, my mind stilled.

My new thought was still prevalent and dominated my mind, repeating itself all the way home from Westwood to Santa Barbara. I heard the same thought, over and over, my personalized God-given mantra: *It's about faith!*

*Romans 14:23: "And he that doubteth is damned if he eat, because he eateth not of faith: for whatsoever is not of faith is sin."*

## The Devil Thing?

I woke up the next morning feeling energetic, feeling great, confident, happy, but confused. I didn't comprehend or believe in the devil theory. *If God wants to heal me in this way, who am I to resist?* I reasoned.

I had had a normal meal. The evidence was conflicting but strong. One thing was certain. It was about faith!

I was starting to eat again. I was feeling my strength returning. *I must be healed,* I thought. *The casting out of devils is healing me.* I had gotten a big gain from something I didn't believe in, something that I thought was crazy!

The casting out of demons may not be so bad, I found myself reconsidering. I thought about going back to the meeting again the following week, and maybe even to Pastor Tim's church on Sunday.

*Luke 9:1: "Then he called His twelve disciples together, and gave them power and authority over all devils, and to cure diseases."*

## Joining the Church

That next Sunday I went to the church, and I was delighted to be there. I didn't get it. I didn't understand it; I didn't care. Whatever was coming out was effective. This was contrary to all of my beliefs up to this point. Even though I didn't buy into the devil concept, I was having some sort of deliverance. I was eating food!

I have since noticed this phenomenon in my personal ministry. You don't have to believe in something to be healed. It's always a shock to me, and an extra joy, when that happens. And it happens a lot. People who do not believe in deliverance, even total nonbelievers in God, get healed all the time! People that do not yet know God get healed. People from all religions, all walks and paths, get healed by Jesus! He is not a respecter of persons!

*Ephesians 6:9: "Neither is there respect of persons with him."*

## Tug of War

I consecrated myself to Pastor Tim's meetings and teachings. I became a regular at these deliverance meetings. All I had to do was show up. Even if I didn't receive personal prayer, the anointing (the energy of the power of the Holy Spirit) had power over my mind! The anointing itself had a power to separate me from my carnal self, lift me up into the spirit and remind me of the truth.

The Holy Spirit is more powerful than any human physical strength; it can override the body. That is why people can be slain, even pass out, by the power of the Holy Spirit.

I was made strong by attending these meetings. The anointing was holding me up! I was able to get a supernatural separation from God's anointing. I was less sensitive to foods, able to go to the meetings, and became less sensitive to some people. But I was not free. I would take a few foods back, but also lose other foods.

I needed information. I was still clueless about how to hold my healing. The devil castings seemed to be either temporary or there was something missing from these procedures.

*1 Corinthians 1:18: "The word of the Cross is the power of God."*

# Chapter 16

## After the Thrill of Eating by Faith

After awhile, when the initial thrill of eating by faith disappeared, I started to feel desperate again. I was once more becoming intolerant to foods. Soon I was subsisting exclusively on organic white rose potatoes.

I contacted another woman I knew who had been spiritually healed through another group of deliverance ministers in Florida. I spoke with Dana, who claimed that she had totally recovered with this new ministry. She gave me their phone number. These ministers were also in the exorcism (deliverance) category of ministry!

I knew that this woman had been ill for years. She had been much sicker than Cynthia; she had nearly died. Dana had gone everywhere to get well; the medical community had given up on her. For years she could not even enter a house. She had been living in the open air in an old broken-down tent. She camped for six years, in all kinds of weather, running from town to town looking for clean air, warm air, safe air, dry air, etc. A perpetual quest for peace and health. She had been trying to stay alive. Barely existing! Through her involvement with this ministry, she had gone from tent living in the isolated sticks of Arizona to a real job in a big corporation in Manhattan. Dana was currently healed and living in a New York City high-rise apartment building.

Very impressive!

*Hebrews 9:12: "By His own blood He entered in
... having obtained eternal redemption for us ..."*

## I Cannot Get There
## (Restoration Ministries)

I decided to telephone the people who had been involved with her healing. We spoke for awhile, and they were kind enough to invite me to participate in their ministry in Green Cove, Florida. I told them that there was no way I could get there. I could not travel. That was out of the question. I could not go into someone else's environment. I was much too sensitive. It was impossible! I explained my situation. They said they would pray about it and call me back.

*Revelation 1:18: "I am he that liveth, and was
dead; and, behold, I am alive forever more ..."*

## Help Is on the Way

They did just that. These ministers were coming to Santa Barbara, to my house, to deliver me! They had prayed and realized the severity of my challenge and felt led by the spirit to come to my home to help me. God was sending to my front door the pastor's wife and a sister, two deliverance ministers. It seemed like exorcisms were becoming a big part of my life, and later would be my calling, but I didn't know that yet. I still didn't believe in devils.

Maybe I never would. Maybe something else was going on. There was, however, an abundance of exorcism-oriented coincidences in my life. Wasn't that true for most people?

*Psalm 121:2: "My help cometh from the Lord,
which made heaven and earth."*

## Rachel and Lynn Arrive

The two deliverance ministers arrived at my door: Rachel and Lynn. I was very excited. I was still extremely sensitive to fumes coming into my home from doors being opened and closed. The opening of a door could, and usually did, allow fumes from the outside to enter. It was a big risk. If enough fumes entered into the living room, I would have to give the room up. I would be unable to live in the house.

There were many nights when I had to relocate from my usual sleeping room — I would be forced to sleep in the bathtub. If enough fumes entered, I would be trapped into living in a tiny bathroom in the back of the house. It would then be necessary to begin a process of weeks of detoxification, trying to exchange good air for bad—a window open here, a door open there, and fans everywhere. I was in one of these air exchange nightmares when these two women arrived. I had to open the door to let them in.

## I Let Them in My Home

They seemed to have entered without adding additional contaminants. I considered this to be a sign from above! We introduced ourselves, and I was very happy to see them. They had unusual beliefs. Sometimes born-again Christians do, we all know this — and these were exorcists!

They immediately began doing strange things in my home with what was left of my possessions. The few items that had survived my illness were now under inspection by these ministers. Everything was being examined for devils. I was being interrogated. My home and my person went under an investigation, a witch-hunt, or in this case a demon hunt.

During my years of isolation, music had become my only solace. According to them, my music was demonic and had to go. Rachel believed that my music could actually be the root of my environmental illness. (Billy Joel was, of course, the devil, and Linda Ronstadt totally possessed.) The two women wanted to build a bonfire in a trash can in my yard. Their intentions were to burn my music along with a few remaining non-biblical books.

I was convinced that this was not my problem, nor would my problem be solved by this intervention. This just wasn't true for me. I knew that I couldn't accept this. I just couldn't give up any more power. I could not bow to any more inauthenticity. I didn't need to have less in my life; I felt that I needed a whole lot more! I found myself getting up from my chair to express myself. I could not allow this invasion go on any longer.

I took a step toward Rachel, to tell both women that this was unacceptable! I wanted them to stop this behavior and get out of my house! I had to let them know that I believed their behavior was compromising my integrity and would not facilitate healing. I perceived that what they were doing was utter self-righteousness!

## Shut Up

I stood up and walked towards the women. Just as I opened my mouth to speak, God intervened and said, *"Sit down, shut up, and go along with them."* I was stopped in my tracks, a change of plans. It was a clear word; I felt it strongly in my heart. It wasn't a small leading of God; it wasn't a revelation. It was a command: *"Shut up. Shut up and go along with them."*

A command from God comes with the exact understanding of what He means and what He wants. It wasn't about the music or the books; it was about going along with them. God had a plan. God had sent them. There were many things that they had to offer me. God was telling me to not get caught up in the small stuff. *"Do not tell them to go. I have sent them and they will be valuable to you."*

I was two feet from Rachel's face, ready to express my good-byes, and had a total change of heart. I abruptly stepped back. The entire energy in the room had changed! The women were aware of it.

I had to offer an explanation for what now looked like very strange behavior on my part. I told them the truth. With a sense of humor, I told them what I was thinking, but admitted, "God has told me to go along with you."

They understood what I was saying. By the look on their faces, they were probably thinking, *She is resisting us but God is intervening, letting her know who we are.* They read it accurately! They, too, were hearing from God.

## We Bonded in the Spirit

The atmosphere had changed in my little wood shack. Peace had entered the room, acceptance had entered the room. We were in total agreement — the kind of agreement that is palpable and changes your perceptions. We were in the will and purpose of God. There was a clarity in the room, a crispness. A glow.

The chemical fumes that had entered into my living room a week ago, that had disturbed me, were gone! The fumes were gone! They had been vanquished when God's plan was acknowledged.

I had left fans all around the room to detoxify the room, but they hadn't dissolved the fumes! They (the exorcists), of course, didn't know this; I hadn't gone into all that with these ministers of the Lord. His vessels were having their own experiences in the peace and blessings of the Holy Ghost!

> Colossians 2:2: "That their hearts might be comforted, being knit together in love ..."

103

## Holy Spirit Intervention

We merged as sisters in the Lord. I was still at this time extremely sensitive to people and their energy. I was able to get close to these ministers without my usual reactions. We all lay down together on my big, nontoxic safe mat. We used this as a piece of furniture, a couch.

They held me in their arms; another glow, another shot of Jesus, still no reactions. I was just going along. I had no answers, but I did have hope. Hope was coming. Who were these amazing women, God's vessels? Who were these deliverance ministers who had the power of God to change the atmosphere in a room?

## Building Trust

I didn't actually go along with the throwing out of my possessions, but I did put everything in a big bag and suggest we leave it in my trunk until I could find someone who might want it. That was between me and the Lord. It was about building trust.

We hung out for a few days. They were instructing me on "the stand." They were imparting Divine wisdom, and I was having trouble getting it. As we drove past a hamburger place, Rachel finally said to me (with a heavy Boston accent), "Look, Juliana, just do it! All you have to do is go in and eat!"

*Doesn't she know*, I wondered, *that someone with my condition can't just eat a hamburger?* I couldn't follow these suggestions. I actually thought that it was cruel that she would mock my inability to eat. It was like telling a cripple, "Just go walk across the street. I'll meet you there on the other side. All you have to do is walk."

## It Is Still a Good Laugh

It was an ongoing joke with us for a long time that Rachel was so cruel that she would tell a starving woman to eat. Eating was, of course, the issue.

I just couldn't do it. After about five days of spending time with the sisters, and going through their deliverance process, Rachel commented, "I think you got this, but if you don't, come back and see us and we'll stand with you."

They invited me to their home in Green Cove, Florida, where they had their ministry and church. We had become good friends, and I was sincerely and joyfully invited to their home.

If I were not successful in my attempts to eat again, I would follow them, and we would all stand together. That was our parting agreement.

# Chapter 17

## Standing on His Victory (Enforcing Grace)

The key word was "stand!" Stand was the missing link! God wanted me to take a stand. I had no stand and that was my problem. I didn't learn at the last deliverance ministry because they weren't teaching the "stand." They were just casting out spirits of deception.

A good exorcist must know that a cast is sometimes only as good as the person's ability to stand. In any miracle healing, we must suspect this and prepare a person for a battle. If the battle is understood, there is no problem. If the battle comes upon a naive and unsuspecting soul, there is great and unnecessary trauma. The fact is that God would prefer us to grow up in Him, increase our faith and hold fast. To stand on His word, His victory, His grace and truth!

> Galatians 5:1: "Stand fast therefore in the
> liberty wherewith Christ hath made us free, and
> be not entangled again with the yoke of bondage."

## Standless in Santa Barbara

About five days after the ministers left, I could not eat again. I called the sisters, standless and desperate. They reiterated that they would stand with me. They asked me to join them in Florida. I didn't know how I would get there. I would have to fly on a plane and sit down next to perfumed, deodorized and scented people. I would have to stay in their home — a normal home with all its normal chemicals and cleaning products! It would be impossible for me to tolerate any of it. I had no choice but to go by faith.

*2 Corinthians 5:7: "For we walk by faith, not by sight."*

## Attacked to Go
## (The Old Creature Kicks and Screams)

I had to prepare my clothes for the trip. I had a huge washer pot outside my house in the backyard. I would put gloves on and several masks, then run out very cautiously during non-traffic hours, when no one else was around, and do my laundry. If any trace of normal detergent or fabric softener touched my clothes, they would be ruined. I would have to dispose of the tainted clothing!

I only had a few rags left, and it was a complicated process to prevent clothes previously washed with detergents from mixing in the same batch with clothes that were boiled with distilled water.

That night in the dryer, there was an "accident," and all the clothes that I had intended to take to Green Cove were ruined. I didn't know what to do. I was up all night, hopeless and crying. I waited until six in the morning and called Rachel. I explained what had happened. "Rachel! My clothes were ruined. I can't travel without clothing. I have nothing, not one shred of clothing that is safe for me to wear!" I shrieked hysterically. "What am I going to do?"

She, too, didn't know what to do. She replied, "Hold on a moment, Juliana."

# Rachel Is Speechless

She turned frantically to her husband, Pastor Hank, and said, "Now what? What should I do? She can't come naked. She has no clothes." She was as confused as I.

"Go back to the phone," Pastor Hank directed, "and pray for her. We are only people, what can we do? The devil has attacked her to keep her from coming here. God will work it out."

Rachel returned to the phone. "Juliana, you are attacked because you are coming here to be healed! Put some clothes on and I'll pray for you."

I did just that. I put the contaminated clothes on and my whole body reacted. I started itching and shaking. I kept the clothing on and picked up the phone. Rachel prayed for me, and the reactions totally stopped.

That was my witness; I knew that God was in it. God was leading me. This edified my faith, and I had new hope. With only the clothes on my back, I would attempt the journey. All I had needed was a small sign from God to be certain that this was His plan, and God had provided just that.

I put the remaining ruined clothing in my suitcase by faith, believing she would pray them on my back when I got there. My suitcase contained one broken-down very old cot to sleep on and clothing I couldn't tolerate. This was not a glamour cruise.

There would be no more casting out of evil! Although many times deliverance ministries will get total healings from the casting out of deceptions, it was my time to stand. God had arranged an entire ministry for me to learn to stand with.

*1 Corinthians 2:5: "That your faith should not stand in the wisdom of man, but in the power of God."*

## The Journey

With new confidence and fully attired in rags, I went to the airport. I felt a flow in the energy. I knew that I was moving in a good direction. I had joy. I was being led by the Spirit. I felt that I was in His purpose. It was a long flight, and it was very late by the time I arrived in Florida.

## Restoration Ministries

I didn't know what to expect. I knew one thing and one thing only: God was in this. Were clothes not prayed on my back for the purpose of this trip? This fact could not be denied! Doubt had lost power to sway me.

I trusted these people. I would obey them. They had gained my absolute confidence. My only unresolved concern had been abated; they were definitely of God, following God, led by God.

They were waiting for me when I got off the plane, right there at the gate. To me, that was a sign that they really cared about me. I was important to them; God's mission had priority in their lives. It was late. The time change made it way past their dinnertime.

I was so spaced out by this time that I was hardly present. I had not flown in an airplane for many years. Car fumes were serious enough for me. An airplane, for an environmentally ill person, was unthinkable — the fumes, the lack of oxygen, the people sitting all around me with perfume, after-shave, etc.!

I had barely escaped an exposure! There was a woman sitting right next to me who was about to spray herself with perfume, a fresher-upper for her arrival.

Quickly, I jumped up in my protective allergic emergency mode. "Please wait! Please wait until I am off the plane before you spray. I am allergic to perfume." I was fortunate she complied. She did, however, give me "the look" … I tightened my air-filter face mask and swallowed my pride.

I had survived the plane trip, and before I knew it I was in a vehicle going to a new residence, someone else's residence. I had not entered another human being's home in more than ten years. Houses had all my allergens in them: carpets, cleansers, laundry detergents, and so much more.

I could not even envision what I would find in the room where I would be staying. I was being taken to the guest apartment above their home, the ministry quarters. The drive was about an hour and a half. Green Cove was a rural town in North Central Florida.

## They Were All Waiting for Me to Eat!

We arrived at their home, and I was in for another surprise. Many of the church members were there in my apartment, waiting for me. They were all part of it. All had prayed and waited to eat; all were excited to meet me, to see me!

I was overwhelmed by so many new faces. I couldn't allow myself to think about what they were wearing or what scents were present. What was the difference? I would soon eat. I had to; I had very little strength left to hang around and ponder food. No, this was it. Eat or fade away.

It was terrifying being in someone else's house! There were at least twelve people there. I had not expected that; I was stunned! Furthermore, I could sense that they were really hungry and though they were serving the Lord, it was late. They had been waiting for me to join them for dinner. After all, this was about the food! We were all hungry.

## Pastor Was Hungry

I saw Pastor glance at his watch. It was 9 p.m., way past his dinner hour. I heard his personal thoughts.

*It's nine now,* he thought, *I wonder how long it's going to take for us to talk Juliana into eating by faith? This could be an all-nighter.*

I turned around and told Pastor Hank what I had heard. "I got it!" I said. "Let's just go eat."

"That's the Holy Ghost," he replied, "letting you into my thoughts!" Pastor smiled as he said that.

Pastor Hank had a way of making everything fun, everything brighter than it was. He enjoyed his life; he fully enjoyed serving His Lord. He was going to fully enjoy this evening and his meal. He was always joyful and had a twinkle in his eye. He was not easily dejected.

"You have hope," he said. "That is good enough for God. Hope brings faith!" He was excited now. The miracle and the meal were nigh, or so he believed.

I was unsure how much faith was involved in that moment on my part. There was a combination of guilt for the folks who were kind enough to wait, a responsibility for their hunger, a hearing of Pastor's thoughts, and necessity.

## No Marathons, Please

We all knew that we could go over this all night long; they could speak faith and pray, and finally, I would have to bite the bullet. Bite some food, anyway! Nothing was going to happen until my action of eating!

They had to get me there; that was their job. I had to lay my life on the line; that was my job! I was there to take my foods back and eat. I felt the tension lift in the air. The folks relaxed. They were breathing easier. Everyone was relieved that this wasn't going to be a marathon.

*John 10:17: "Therefore doth my Father love me,*
*because I lay down my life, that I might take it up again."*

## The Decision

The minute that I made the decision to go ahead and eat, my mind went into a combined state of fear and euphoria. I knew I was going to do this (eat by faith), yet I couldn't really feel anything. The decision had within it such anxiety that it put me into almost a drugged state. I could only describe it as euphoric terror — high anxiety in a numbed state, a mental paralysis. I knew that this was it! I was going to do this, make it or break it. It was Jesus or bust. Pastor was right. I had hope. I hoped I would live!

## Food Is not God

We went to a small Southern greasy buffet restaurant. Selections were very minimal for someone who was used to eating organic foods. There was nothing organic, nothing from Atkins, nothing macrobiotic, nothing plain. Even items as simple as steamed vegetables were absent from the menu. To even suggest such options would be absurd.

I can only assure you, in retrospect, that if I saw those same foods today, I would pass. I didn't actually see them. I was too disconnected from my body to feel or see. I filled my plate with a smorgasbord of Southern-fried junk food and ate. I did not choose food or evaluate what was better or worse. I was in a food category that I had never known before.

Many of these foods I could not even recognize. I ate and ate. What was the difference? I would live or die. More food, more faith; more faith, more grace. I needed all the grace I could get. I had pies, ice cream, and the forbidden yeast breads, with butters and jams.

I ate. I tasted nothing. I felt nothing. I ate more. It was clear to all that my appetite was not the problem!

## When I Realized What I Had Eaten!

It soon became apparent that I would survive the meal. Later, when we all returned to the restaurant again and I was able to see the food that I had eaten that night, it became a joke with us — the cosmic joke that my first meal, as far as I was concerned, was the most allergic group of foods on earth itself. God had brought me to the perfect place to confront the worst food groups on the planet.

## God Is God

I continued to eat the unidentifiable Southern-fried greasy junk foods and lived on Dairy Queen for six weeks. I gained sixty-five pounds and ended up more than twice my previous weight. I blossomed in great health.

That was my personal expose' on the illusion of food. Food had become an idol! I had given my power to food, and I was taking it back. God was showing me the powerlessness of foods as healer. My beliefs about foods were being broken. Food was not God. God was God.

## Faith Is not Just One Carrot

In the busting of a con, a mental deception of the carnal mind, the ante must be upped. That is where faith comes in. One must identify and defy the idol; tear down the strong man (the lie), the erroneous belief that has exalted itself above the knowledge and power of God. This is the bringing down of strongholds and every high thing that exalts itself against the knowledge of God. (2 Corinthians 10:4-5)

The best way to do this is to up the ante, to demonstrate your authority in Christ. Make your point via action! For example, if I am allergic to carrots, if I am unable to eat and digest one carrot, I will get sick. If I eat two carrots, I will get sicker. If I eat three, I will probably get even sicker. If I eat twenty carrots, I have made my point! I have enforced my Grace; I have established my dominion. I have said by my actions of faith that carrots have no power over me.

We as believers of God have misinterpreted what faith is, and that deception has kept the body of Christ out of its rightful authority. Miracle faith is upping the ante and demonstrating the grace and power of God. Miracle faith may include a little "spiritual retaliation."

> *Isaiah 35:4: "Behold, your God will come with vengeance, even God with a recompence: he will come and save you."*

## Wrong Identification

We have given our power to physical identification. We must take it back. This belief that we have bought that we are our body is a con of the old nature. With this one deception, we become prone to a lifetime of illusion.

Until we spiritualize our perceptions, we will always be victims of the flesh. This is a technique of your personally inherited generational principalities (old seed consciousness) to keep you from your proper identification. If you find out that you have been given dominion over your body and thoughts, you reign. No more sickness, pains, or surrendering to "beliefs of old age."

I am not talking about some pie-in-the-sky afterlife promise, but right here on earth now.

The Lord did not give you the victory for your afterlife. He gave it to you for your current life, right here and right now. This very minute. *This is where you need it — today on earth!*

> *Galatians 2:20: "I am crucified with Christ: nevertheless I live: yet not I, but Christ liveth in me: and the life which I now live in the flesh I live by the son of God, who loved me, and gave himself for me."*

# Chapter 18

## Tax the Devil

The type of faith that will expedite Divine Healing is the faith for "Divine Retaliation." Always take a little something extra. *Tax the devil.* Let evil know not to mess with you!

You are the King's seed. If you want to grow in an accelerated manner and get more of God and His power, retaliate! Evil will learn to think twice before messing with you! You will be training your own flesh to obey you.

This is called bringing the flesh under subjection. This is a very real biblical way to sanctify flesh from spirit.

*1 Corinthians 9:27: "But I keep under my body, and bring it into subjection: lest that by any means, when I have preached to others, I myself should be castaway."*

Retaliation faith brings the power and grace of God. If you did nothing, knew absolutely nothing, and just kept walking by faith, taking your personal land, God Himself would raise your consciousness to His. If you never studied anything or read anything, but simply understood the authority granted you in the blood of Jesus and the grace of God, greater things would you be doing than the Lord Himself.

## Sanctification

Sanctification is not a religious experience. It is a lifestyle of authority in Christ. You can live under subjection to the old creature, even if you are not aware of it. That would be living in denial. This is a victimized, powerless lifestyle, one where the mind is above the spirit. The spirit is oppressed. Medication can't change that. Without spiritual oppression, there are no illnesses. Without spiritual oppression, there are no bad days, no depressions, no loneliness, no heartbreak.

The fruit of the spirit is love, joy, peace, power, purpose, divine health, dominion on this earth. The fruit of the old nature (carnality) is death, the law of sin and death being its master. Sanctification is survival.

The resurrection and sanctification power of Jesus Christ on this earth is your only weapon for separating yourself from mortal circumstance. I am not talking about eternal life. I am not pontificating lofty spiritual morality. I am talking about surviving on a day-to-day basis.

> Galatians 5:22: *"But the fruit of the Spirit is love, joy, peace, longsuffering, gentleness, goodness, faith, meekness, temperance: against such there is no law."*

## A Knock on My Door

After the initial shock of eating the junk food and surviving, and before I could get into too much inner deliberation, there was a knock on my door. I was in a strange state. I was not having food reactions, which was amazing, but I was having shock reactions.

I thought that I would feel great once I had the victory of eating! But I was learning that when you are as terrified as I was, you feel nothing. It would take me awhile to feel again. Fear had me numb. You can feel fear and still walk in faith.

Don't let religious mentalities take you out of the faith game with self-righteous beliefs of "you can't have faith and fear at the same time."

I have noticed that people who make those kinds of comments have never stepped out in faith and have no testimony. Faith is in your action; if fear is a reaction, more action will wear it down. Fear will pass as you are not immobilized by focusing on it. Keep moving.

> *1 Corinthians 4:20: "For the kingdom*
> *of God is not in word, but in power."*

## We're Going to the Mall

Knocking at my door bright and early the next morning—not giving my opposition time to counteract their good works—were four of the sisters. They were excitedly waiting for me to participate in our next adventure! Sister Lynn announced the plan. "We're going to the mall! You have no clothes. Today you will wear normal clothes, new clothes. God wants you out of your rags!"

## Are They Crazy?

*Are they crazy?* I wondered. I hadn't attempted to buy a new piece of clothing in ten years. I couldn't wear clothes with chemical dyes and synthetic fibers. They were living in a dream world.

Yet, I felt I couldn't deny them. How could I? I was in their home. They had been so kind to me, they were there for me. I had never experienced this kind of devotion before in my life. There was no money involved. Their motives were totally unselfish and Godly.

I knew that this would be a wasted trip to the mall, but, as a courtesy for their kindness and respect for their time and faith, I would go along with them.

## Why Not Just Walk on Water?

I was sick and nauseated on the way to the mall. The car fumes alone were debilitating to me! They really believed that I would buy new clothes and wear them! Brand new materials! Wouldn't I be wearing them now if it were that easy? I was in a mental battle; my old nature was not going to relinquish more land than absolutely necessary.

The carnal mind wanted to create doubt with its negative line of thinking: *Just eat, just put clothes on your back. It's the just-walk-on-water attitude again! Wait till they see you can't even walk into a clothing store.*

## I Walk into a Real Mall

I went blindly along, without expectations, no hope or faith in this adventure at all. We all walked together into a Contempo Casuals clothing store. I was very aware of all the new fabrics throwing off their scents. The perfume on the saleswoman had me reeling. My eyes were on the new carpet; the combined fragrances of all the new materials were overpowering to me!

I was ready to bolt, just run out of the store, and then suddenly, just in time to arrest my run, the anointing of the Holy Spirit fell upon me. It clobbered me so strongly that, instead of going for the nearest door, I changed my direction and my attitude! I turned around and looked at Sister Lynn and said with excitement, "I really am going to get new clothes today, aren't I?"

I believed it now! I felt it now.

It was true! They weren't pushing limits; they knew stuff. Imagine, here in a little hidden town in the South, were folks who knew the deep things of God. Where I lived in Southern California, I knew of no one who was as informed about these advanced ways of the Lord.

## First Time in a Decade

For the first time in a decade, I began trying on new clothes. I was shaking like a leaf and severely reacting to the toxic materials. I knew the one important thing I needed to know to maintain my faith: God Himself was in it!

The atmosphere in the store had changed, and suddenly I was in the presence of Glory. The Holy Spirit was in the room, lifting me up! I was breathing as a spirit, as if the Lord Himself were breathing for me; my breath was effortless, fuller. All my senses had been transformed; my breath was deepened into a spirit's position. I was inhaling and exhaling fully, from an area deep behind my heart. I was elevated above my problems, supernaturally. I was in the midst of a move of God, seeing through the eyes of the spirit, through the eyes of faith. My emotions had been translated from flesh to higher ground. Even my skin tone had been changed. I was vibrant! God was meeting my step; these devoted servants had led me into this serendipity.

My spirit was ready and righteously indignant at having taken this abuse for so long. My heart was grieved at having been deprived of all my human rights — my peace, my comfort, decent clothing, food and companionship.

## A Literal Standing with Me

Sister Lynn stood close by. "Just let that shaking happen with your body," she said. "It's the devil trying to wear you down. It will pass. You're standing now."

The sisters were on both sides of me — one on the left, one on the right. They had me in between them. They were truly standing with me—they were practically holding me up! My body was rocking; I was in a state of virtual seizure. "Don't focus on your lying symptoms," Sister Lynn kept reminding me.

As I allowed the clothing to remain on my body and ignored the lying symptoms, God honored me with another wave of His anointing. Another jolt of Jesus, another assurance from the Holy Spirit that I had entered into the Kingdom of God. I was surrounded by Glory. I was being upheld, blessed, and healed. God was acknowledging and responding to my faith. God was with me. I was elated!

> *Psalm 3:3: "But thou, O Lord, are a shield to me;*
> *my glory, and the lifter up of mine head."*

## I Was Taken by Surprise

I looked at Lynn and repeated with surprise, "I'm actually going to get new clothes today!"

I believed it now. I would get new clothes this day! I started getting very excited. Thrilled! I was actually wearing new clothes. This was incredible! I was taken totally by surprise. I would look like a civilized human being again.

I had dealt with my strange appearance by avoiding it. I never looked in a mirror; it was too weird. I didn't recognize myself, nor did I care; vanity was not the issue, my mind was on survival. It would take me awhile to experience the luxury of vanity again. A long while.

## A Hamburger Joint

We continued on with our outing. The sisters wanted to have lunch in the mall. Imagine, a real hamburger joint! I would eat a hamburger. That was the very same food that Rachel had teased me about in Santa Barbara. I was starting to get it! I was, of course, the same person here as I was in Santa Barbara, only now I was not starving.

I've said the same words to clients in my ministry. I encourage them to just eat! They look at me like I must be out of my mind. Then there is the moment that they get it. They get the revelation of divine retaliation and they eat! They always have a healing move of God. I've never seen it fail.

*1 Corinthians 1:9: "God is faithful, by whom ye were called unto the fellowship of his Son Jesus Christ our Lord."*

In my situation, *I was simply calling the bluff of deception, backing up evil forces, upping the ante by faith.* To see God meet me in this way was a new and very exciting experience.

## I Am Fine and Full

My stomach was full, and I was wearing new clothes! This may sound primitive to you, but for me, survival was a big deal.

*Deuteronomy 32:43: "Rejoice all ye nations, for he will avenge the blood of his servants, and will render vengeance to his adversaries, and will be merciful unto his land, and unto his people."*

# Chapter 19

## Round Three

I had been joyful, feeling positive about moving on, my unlived life ahead of me. I enjoyed my new family, attended the church, fellowshipped with my brothers and sisters and had a grand time. All had been going well; my reactions were minimal. I had been eating and living large.

## A Counterattack

On the fifth day, everything changed! I was down, bloated, paralyzed with constricting muscle pain and fatigue, itching from head to toe, mentally catatonic. I had begun to react to the foods I'd eaten. It seemed as if all the junk foods had caught up with me!

That was the story that the flesh wanted me to buy. That was the presented con of the carnal mind and, of course, the corresponding symptoms! My healing party was over. I was afraid to eat again. I knew these kinds of reactions too well. My joy was oppressed. Gone! My good life was over! After hearing of these attacks, my new family immediately "sent in the troops."

## The Family of God Arrives

The troops arrived, and there was much Bible reading and prayer — rounds of scripture, sisters taking turns and reading what they felt led to share.

I was lying on my old broken-down cot—down for the count. I said nothing. I looked like a corpse. I had nothing to contribute. The sisters continued to read from the Bible and pray. I was lifeless.

My generational mind was on a tangent, freaking out, getting scared and negative. *"This insanity isn't working. You're ready to die. You can no longer eat that garbage."* These were the type of attack thoughts I was hearing.

Lynn continued reading from the Bible and began to repeat one sentence over and over: "Jesus is alive."

Everyone ceased praying. She had it! We all knew that. She was the one; God was using her. She repeated the same phrase, "Jesus is alive. Jesus is alive."

There was silence. Then, on the next "Jesus is alive," from her spirit to mine, the Holy Spirit intervened.

She kept saying it over and over. "Jesus is alive!" Somehow God used that sentence to impart something into my spirit. I received it, and in that moment I knew exactly what God wanted me to do.

## I Got It

I told the sisters that I knew what I needed to do. It was too late to start that night. The sisters agreed and left. I slept through the night, and the next morning, I got up and intuitively changed the way I would have ordinarily released an attack or an oppression.

In my days as a psychologist and an emotional release therapist, I would have released an oppression emotionally, through screaming, yelling; pushing it out on a feeling level. We called this an anger release. It is actually the spirit of self-justification throwing you a bone, allowing your soul to release its anger.

The impostor knows that all it has to do is think the same thought back in your mind, and you would need to release anger again and again! The impostor knows that that thought creates feelings. First the thought, then the emotions. In addition — for the spiritually naive, if you will go for it — as a bonus for the weakened spirit, it might throw in some extra painful and distracting lying symptoms.

That was what I was personally experiencing in my current warfare. God wanted to teach me how to take my spirit above my emotions and thoughts. I was learning how to stand against my mind with my spirit. My spirit had to reign over my flesh. My mind could no longer be controlled by my flesh.

I was born again. My carnal mind was predestined to be dominated. My spirit was given this authority by Jesus Christ. I had to learn how to appropriate it. I had to know that this power was available to me. Even as a baby in Him, a new Christian, sanctification was available to me. It was mine.

*Hebrews 10:14: "For by one offering he hath perfected for ever them that are sanctified."*

## The Next Morning

I awakened in the same shape that I had been in the day before — sick and miserable. I remembered the night before, and the word that God had given me. I knew I had to implement it. I crawled out of my cot.

## The Plan of the Law of Sin and Death

The enemy of God had a plan for the rest of my trip. Its plan was to take God's healing from me, to take everything I had gained, to create doubt and unbelief, to leave me angry at not being met and to blame God! The law of sin simply refused to give up its victim so easily. Had I not bowed?

The law of sin thought that it had a right to control my mind. It lodged its hate and fear in my back; it loved to strike my back, locking my entire pelvis. I had pain from my lower back all the way down my legs, and I could not turn in either direction. I was stiffened by this counterattack to my attempts at moving ahead. It was using food to justify itself and its evil, trying to distract me from its ungodly plan, lest it be discovered.

And, as usual, finding a scapegoat to blame for its subterfuge actions: Southern-fried greasy junk food—this is what it wanted me to believe.

This one deception alone could kill me or certainly take me out of any future power. One good lie, one con bought could destroy my life! Its evil point was this: *It's over. You can't eat food. Go home!*

## I Am Not My Body

I knew that I was not my body. I was His vessel, and I was here for a purpose. I had received a word from Sister Lynn. Evil did not want me to accomplish this word. This word would be fatal for its planned spiritual warfare. The implementing of this word would take me over the edge and empower me!

The opposition wanted me on my way, pronto. The impostor wanted me out of Green Cove, away from these ministers and back in isolation. The impostor was getting nervous. The tables were turning!

*Psalm 23:5: "Thou preparest a table in the presence of mine enemies: thou anointest my head with oil; my cup runneth over."*

## God's Plan

I was being led to wage a war! I didn't look much like a warrior that morning. But Lynn's word had spoken to my heart. I knew what I had to do, I just didn't know how. I had to get upheld in Christ. I needed a battery charge!

## The Battle between the Flesh and Spirit

I unpacked the little notebook of scriptures that I had collected under the instruction of the ministers a few weeks back. I had traveled with these scriptures; I had read them on the plane. They were scriptures of empowerment and who I was in Christ. I had selected them by the leading of the Holy Spirit.

> *Esther 4:14: "... and who knoweth whether thou art come to the kingdom for such a time as this?"*

I had no idea how to do this, but I was willing. Lynn's word had inspired me. I just didn't know what to do. I was lethargic, numb and powerless!

I had to get alive in Christ. I needed a little resurrection power. I had to come up in my spirit, bring my flesh under subjection ... there would have to be a changing of the "guard," a switch of authority.

> *Galatians 5:17: "For the flesh lusteth against the Spirit, and the Spirit against the flesh."*

It was the carnal mind versus the spirit of God. I would learn to call this a righteousness rebuttal.

# Chapter 20

## Jesus Is Alive

"Jesus is alive" was the word that God had imparted into my spirit. "Jesus is alive" was spoken from the Holy Ghost, given from one heart to another. When Sister Lynn had spoken that truth, God had given me a vision, a revelation, an understanding that there was a great purpose in that word for me. Sister Lynn felt it, and that's why she kept repeating it. I had to become alive, resurrected in Christ. Did He not live in me?

I had His life. I was born again and had the Holy Spirit. That was not my issue. My issue was that my flesh didn't like it. Flesh dies hard, kicks and screams. God was giving me an opportunity for empowerment. I was being led to confront my predestined battle. I would call this battle; I would be the aggressor.

*Romans 6:19: "I speak after the manner of men because of the infirmity of your flesh: for as ye have yielded your members servants to uncleanness and to iniquity unto iniquity; even so now yield your members servants to righteousness unto holiness."*

## I Pick Up the Sword

*Ephesians 6:17: "And take the helmet of salvation, and the sword of the Spirit, which is the word of God."*

I had to listen to what the "enmity" was confessing, what I had been buying. I had to lie back a little and get an understanding of my opponent. I pulled myself to a standing position.

*"You can't move, let alone fight,"* the devil said. *"You are totally de-energized; go back and lie down."*

I felt that thought hit me—felt it hit my body. This was getting interesting. When I watched or listened with a separation, with a focused awareness of the thought, with an understanding that this thought was my opponent, I could observe and feel the connection!

I took a hit! The Lord was educating me! Yes I see, Lord! I was in a boxing match. It was a moment-to-moment warfare; a hostile thought was a blow, a deception was a body shot, a low blow. As soon as I received that thought, I was drained, totally weakened. The carnal mind was being used to create energy shifts! My own carnal mind's thinking could create a symptom in my body! Deceptive thought was oppressing me!

My body was responding to thought! "The power of Christ rests in me," I retorted.

I heard no response. I spoke up. "The power of Christ rests in me. I have all power over you!"

I felt a little bow by the enemy. I had given my first spiritual hit. I had given a blow!

*"The power of Christ you can't eat,"* the devil replied directly to me, its intended victim.

My enemy was enraged, we were on, and we both knew exactly where we stood! The generational mind wasn't hiding anymore with little threats, thus creating hidden fears and anxieties. My opposition was speaking plain, throwing its hate right at me. If I knew what was up, it would come to the foreground, be direct. Provoked. I had provoked evil!

## I Grabbed My Little Notebook

My carnal mind was saying, *You can't eat! You are swollen and sick! You'll never eat again. It's over. You've lost all the foods you've gained.*

I began to fight back, this time with my spirit. My spirit had become alive! My spirit automatically fought against the thoughts and beliefs of the carnal mind.

"I eat by faith," I replied. "If it's not from faith, it's sin."[1] Boom! A little hit.

The devil came back, as strong as ever. "You can't eat, you can't digest food. It's over. You are weak!"

"Louder," the Holy Spirit was directing me. "Louder!"

The impostor continued to taunt me. "You're weak."

"I am weak?" I took my identity back. "In Him I live and breathe and have my being. How can I be weak? I am a dead woman; my life is dead and I am hid in Christ!"[2]

A little resistance, but I was now able to see my opponent's reaction to my words. My words also created a reaction; my words had power! My words knocked it down a little, not a total knockout, but they were able to bring my adversary under subjection!

The strange thing was it was all in the moment. If I tried to just rap scriptures, I was ineffective. I would not be retorting, replying, catching it, busting the con—I would be babbling neurotically.

I found that there was no power in neurotic babbling. That was religion! That was the law justifying itself. I responded with truth, in the moment. I was led to reply to error with truth and authority.

I was able to feel the emotions that it was throwing at me and separate myself. I saw a lot of fear. I could feel and see fear diminish, see it bow when I spoke God's truth. This deception also had life, had a mentality, a will, a purpose. Its purpose was in opposition to God. Always the direct opposite!

To read things in the Bible and believe them is one thing, but to experience the battle that the Bible discusses—to see its absolute truth and validity in action—was incredible!

1 Romans 14:23
2 Colossians 3:3

## A Righteous Rebuttal

"You are dying," the devil said.

"The spirit is life because of righteousness,"[3] I replied. Boom! I gave a blow! A strong one!

I went on a rebuttal roll; I was empowered by my own expression. My own truth, coming out of my mouth, had power to elevate me! I was being uplifted by expressing words of authority.

"The Lord my God upholds the righteous. I am the Righteousness of God in Christ, called with a Holy calling, taking nothing for myself!"[4]

"You are sick, you are crippled, you are finished, helpless. Look at you," error lied back.

"I walk in the Spirit; I do not fulfill the lusts of the flesh.[5] I am far above all power and might and dominion.[6] The weapons of my warfare are not carnal, but mighty through God to the pulling down of strongholds; casting down imaginations, and every high thing that exalteth itself against the knowledge of God."[7]

I was then able to watch fear grip my body, as if it had tendrils, holding onto its prey like a wolf with a carcass in its mouth.

The devil threw a cramp in my stomach. "Look at you," it remarked. "You couldn't eat today; you will get worse."

"I am not my stomach," I replied, "for the Kingdom of God is not meat and drink, but righteousness, peace, and power in the Holy Ghost![8] As far as the east is from the west, am I from you.[9] My life is dead, dead, being born again not of corruptible seed but of incorruptible seed by the word of God."[10]

A score on the spirit's side; the old nature didn't like the seed acknowledgment. The seed warfare had an extra power. The opposition took a blow there ... I went up a little, my first real

3  Romans 8:10
4  Isaiah 41:13
5  Galatians 5:16
6  Ephesians 1:21

7  2 Corinthians 10:4–5
8  Romans 14:17
9  Psalm 103:12
10  1 Peter 1:23

sign of light. I was starting to feel encouraged. I was losing a sense of time!

The battle was verbal; I was speaking to it outside myself, as if there were another person in the room. The battle got loud. We were fighting, "duking it out."

Deception interrogated me. "Who do you think you are? Are you insane? You still can't eat. You can't go anywhere. You are very, very sick."

"You are sick," I said, the volume of my voice raised by the Holy Spirit. "Do not confuse yourself with me. I am authentic; you are a counterfeit, an impostor. I am the regenerated spirit.

"A renewed woman, all power hath been given unto me.[11] The spirit knoweth all things.[12] The Kingdom of heaven suffereth violence, and the violent take it by force.[13] I have boldness to enter into the holiest by the blood of Jesus[14] … that's who I am; His righteousness is who I am."

I then began to feel my true feelings—not emotions, but spiritual fruits. The righteous indignation, which only comes from the battle, was being developed. I started to come up in it, to become it.

"How dare you undermine me! I am far, far above all principality and power, and might and dominion.[15] I have been given dominion on this earth.[16] I am separate, sanctified, saved."[17]

"You sanctified?" the devil responded. "You're a mess."

I countered. "By one blood offering He hath perfected forever them that are sanctified."[18]

A big blow, blood and seed. It became apparent that the blood and the seed had an extra power in the spiritual realm.

Things began to change; I began to feel it. I had my helper with me. The Holy Ghost was taking over. I had made myself available and agreed with God's perceptions. "His blood hath

11  Matthew 28:8
12  1 Corinthians 2:11
13  Matthew 11:12
14  Hebrews 10:19

15  Ephesians 1:21
16  Ephesians 1:21
17  1 Corinthians 6:11
18  Hebrews 10:14

translated me, I am redeemed, forgiven, according the riches of His Grace."[19]

"I don't listen to you," I went on, even louder now. "If I live after the flesh, I will die; for the flesh sets its desire against the spirit and the spirit against the flesh.[20] I wrestle not against flesh and blood but against principalities rulers of this world, against spiritual wickedness in high places.[21] The first man is of the earth; the second man is the Lord from heaven.[22] The first man Adam was made a living soul; the last Adam was made a quickening spirit."[23]

"That's me alive in Christ, a quickening spirit, quickened together with Christ."[24]

"Hallelujah! Amen. Jesus is alive! I am not sick, oppressed, weak; I am alive in Christ that the power of Christ may rest upon me."[25]

## The Good Fight of Faith

It went on like that for about an hour and fifteen minutes, fighting the good fight between my carnal self (the old man) and my spiritual self (the new creature in Christ) until my spirit came out on top. I was transformed into being my spirit woman as I expressed my true nature. I was speaking myself into experiencing the power of the word that the Holy Spirit had delegated to my Sister Lynn.

With every hostile suggestion that my carnal thought would express, I retorted with a scripture from my little notebook. It didn't happen right away, not at the first word barrage, not at the first rebuttal, but soon *I was able to see the thought rise up and the scripture attack*!

It was like watching a boxing match. I would be hit, attacked, take a thought blow, be pushed down mentally, emotionally,

19  Ephesians 1:7
20  Galatians 5:17
21  Ephesians 6:12
22  1 Corinthians 15:47
23  1 Corinthians 15:45
24  Ephesians 2:5
25  2 Corinthians 12:9

physically. Then I would strike back with a scripture— louder, bigger, a counterpunch.

## It Was a Battle Led by God

I wasn't just throwing out words, but waiting ... watching ... hearing ... and responding.

I had to have the final say, word by word, thought by thought, as the battle raged. I had to be present in His Spirit, in His moment, in His Kingdom, like any great conqueror.[26] I had to know that I had the victory!

I was just enforcing His Grace with His word. His word would perform what it set out to do. It could not possibly return void.[27] The Master would back His word. I had won the "war of words." The carnal thought had bowed to my spiritual authority.

The carnal mind had to bow to spiritual truths and the authority of Christ. All I had to do was pick up the sword and wage the battle, the rebuttal ... It was a strange battle!

## I Gave Deception a Beating

I had watched the word annihilate deception. This was not a conversation. I was giving deception a whipping, a beating. I was kicking butt in the spiritual realm. I was piggybacking a victory that the Lord had won two thousand years ago.

I had a reason to be indignant: how dare the devil try to take something from me that had been freely given! Glory to God in the Highest!

> Romans 13:4: "For He is the minister of God to thee for good.
> But if thou do that which is evil, be afraid; for he beareth
> not the sword in vain: for he is a minister of God,
> a revenger to execute wrath upon him that doeth evil."

26  Romans 8:37
27  Isaiah 55:11

# Chapter 21

## The Sword Is Not Religion

There are people who listen to the word all day on tape and memorize every scripture, but when they get sick, they run to the doctor! It was not that kind of a battle. It was about faith in His word, faith in the truth. You can pick up any scripture that your heart knows is true for you today, right now—and slay deception!

I had nothing — a little notebook, a tiny little pad the size of an address pocket book! I picked it up in the moment, in the battle, in the land, in the appointed turf of the battle. There is a territory where you go to take back your land, a spiritual territory—the "spot" where you will be empowered. It is there that God will instruct and do the rest ... willingness is all that is necessary.

Not being in the moment in a battle, or using the word out of the moment, is a way to be disempowered, a trap. It then becomes a planned battle, an agenda, a war that is not led by God—a war that you can lose!

> Galatians 5:18: "But if ye be led of
> the Spirit, ye are not under the law."

This is the battle that will keep you in the spirit. To not identify and partake in this battle is to be suffering needlessly. *Enforce your identity in Christ.*

## The Agenda Is the Law

Using the word as a declaration out of the moment is a mental battle. Mental ascent will not create sanctification. Only an "in the moment" battle has spiritual power and is deliverance of the heart, mind, body and soul!

Stay away from religious perceptions of the Bible. You will lose the very power that you need. Do not let error turn your sword into condemnation. This is your very vital weapon. Protect yourself from religious interpretations derived from generational guilt and victimization. These undermining interpretations are the exact opposite of the grace of God. *Beware the guilt-ridden and evil projections of the impostor in your own mind and in the carnal minds of others who may be oppressed in this scheme.* Sin consciousness does not glorify God or empower you!

Remember at all times that love fulfills the law. If you are being taught the law without love and fellowship, the teaching is probably rooted in deception.

The generational law and its self-righteousness would like to make the heart of man an endangered species. This is a spirit of mind control. It can be discerned by the headache or oppression you get in its presence. It is intolerable to the heart. Don't fall for it!

*Romans 2:20: "An instructor of the foolish, a teacher of babes, which hast the form of knowledge and of the truth in the law."*

## Babeland

If you are in a congregation that is, in most part, oppressed, you are probably in Babeland! Babeland is a very dangerous place. It is a place where the curse thrives; it has full reign in the law. In Babeland, there is a focus on works, a constant and subtle undermining of the finished work of the Cross of Calvary and the sufficiency of His grace.

Not only will you not get healed in Babeland, there are actually more disabled people in Babeland than out on the street! There are more healthy and mentally sound folks outside of these oppressive religious settings, just living in the world. It is a natural outcome of the laws that have been set in place, laws that control the universe. If there is less law (less curse), there are more blessings!

Remember always the simplicity that is in Christ. What Christ did for you was to separate you from the Law of Sin and Death (sin consciousness) and translate you into the Perfect Law of Liberty. By one blood offering, you have become the righteousness of God in Christ, transformed from your old nature to be the spirit person God created—the seed of Christ. *Do not allow the carnal mind of man to make the cross of Christ null and void in your life.*

The Lord is about to shake Babeland up and separate the righteous from the flesh. This inauthentic and shallow move of the flesh will be exposed and left behind in God's new authentic move of the spirit.

The new move will be of uncompromising integrity with demonstrations of supernatural power. The Lord is not going to entrust His supernatural power to the pursuers of personal fame and finances. *The spirit of self-exaltation is about to take a blow on earth. Its long and powerful reign shall be diminished!*

In Babeland, you are always the condemned sinner; there is no separation of identities. You are never taught who you are in Christ. You are never taught how to bring your carnal mind, thoughts and body under subjection. The focus in Babeland is usually on an individual, a man or woman, a personality, not on the Cross of Christ and the power of God. Sermons are prepared in advance, and there is a lot of worldly talk. People talk about themselves too much! You are constantly told to pray more, read more, tithe more, do something more … that is Babeland. These churches are not led by the Holy Spirit of God but by carnal agenda. Many of these religious churches thrive on the same dysfunctional codependent behavior that God wants you delivered from.

Stop giving your power to man! It is idolatry at its finest! It will inhibit your freedom and blessings in Christ.

If you are not being edified and instructed to step out in faith and take your personal land, you are probably in works. You might be in a repetitive generational dysfunction! *Instead of being transformed, you could be repeating and reliving your unhealed past with a new religious family! Remember, your grace is by faith, and faith is of action.* Works (trying to get to God without faith) is the fastest way I know of to thwart the grace of God. It creates an instant disconnection. This place of works and disempowerment can be felt and identified by a lack of peace, neediness, and constant confusion. It is based in our most primal fear: the "fear of" separation from our creator.

> *Romans 2:18: "For the wrath of God is revealed from heaven against all ungodliness and unrighteousness of men, who hold the truth in unrighteousness."*

## The Word of God Is in Your Heart (Proverbs 3:3)

The Word of God, God's word, anointed in the Holy Spirit, has the final say on this planet. His word is the pinnacle of His power. There are other areas in life where we must become aware of words.

## Thoughts Are Words

Your thoughts, your very own thoughts, are affecting your heart. Thoughts received are the condition of your heart.

## Words and Thoughts

This is very freeing. You can control the energy of your day by speaking righteous words, and by simply not receiving undermining words. Words that are not honest and true can, if received, lower your power.

You, as a trained and capable warrior of God, would never be undermined by doubt or error. Your spirit is aware of the word battle and has a heightened sensitivity to it. It has a gifted and Godly hearing capacity to discern, identify and not receive any and all victimizing words.

## Guard Your Heart!

You would never allow yourself to be verbally abused! If someone were to attack you and say, "You are an idiot, a worthless slob disconnected from God and going nowhere," you would vehemently disagree. You would vigorously respond; you would not receive such a lie. Words of disempowerment can be very subtle in the spiritual realm. Once you begin to "hear" and respond appropriately in spirit and truth, you will never be disempowered again.

> *Ephesians 4:15: "Speaking our truth with love we grow up in all aspects of Him."*

## Word War

Knowledge of the "word war" will change your entire life. You can go from victimization to total victory, total dominion, with a few words, as I did in the previous story. "Word" power can be applied to every situation in your life.

> *Romans 10:17: "Faith comes from hearing and hearing by the word of God."*

## Inner Boundaries

Bust the con of your flesh and set an inner boundary to the words of the old creature perpetually trying to make a comeback in your life. It is your life — you, the spirit person. A life bought and paid for by the blood of Jesus. All power hath been given unto you. Mortify the deeds of the flesh. Life in the spirit is death to the flesh. Mortify!

John 11:25: "I am the resurrection and the life; he that believeth on me, though he were dead, yet he shall live."

# Chapter 22

## Your Power Is in the New Moment

Denial means simply not being present in the new moment — not hearing and responding to the new words. You do not need to go back and confront old times. Come into a new moment with your situations and hear, hear, hear! Listen to the words being spoken in your mind, and respond from your authentic self. You will find that all your power is right there in the moment.

As we take land, we step out in faith, thereby bringing our idols under subjection. We become naturally upheld in the spirit. Your spiritual hearing and power will be increased via faith. You, the spirit person in the dispensation of grace, would never allow error to oppress your heart.

How great is our salvation that God has given us word control and a sword to enforce His ultimate Word over all situations. We have the last and final say over all deception!

I had just had my first "word victory."

## What's Going on Up There?

It had been a noisy battle. The Pastor and his wife had come home and heard the commotion. They had called in the troops to see what was going on. Sister Lynn was sent over to investigate. The timing was perfect; I had just about wrapped up the battle. I was praising in my victory. Sister Lynn was knocking aggressively when I opened the door. She looked at me and rapidly assessed the situation. "You look like you've just won a battle."

I was still praising the Lord. "Lynn, I am higher than I have ever been before in my life! I have been given a weapon. I have been empowered; I used the sword, the sword of the Spirit!

"I used it, and God met me! I feel great. All my pains are gone; my mind is stilled. I have great energy and strength. I know that I can digest food. I know that I can eat anything now!" I was ready for some junk food, a good Southern-fried greasy banquet and some Dairy Queen for dessert. All my food concerns and reactions had vanished. I had conquered them with the word! Hallelujah!

*Revelation 1:16: "And out of his mouth went a sharp two-edged sword."*

## Dancing with Jesus

Lynn understood; we began praising God together. We rejoiced together in my victory! Lynn suggested that we share my testimony with the rest of the ministry. They were working at the church office that morning. We walked over and told my tale of victory. The entire staff gathered around and joined us in praise. They totally ceased all of their actions to glorify God! We all congregated together and praised the Lord for over an hour. It was a joyous day.

That was the best day of my life so far. I was dancing with Jesus! This paled any experience that I had had to date. There was no man, no party, no financial security, nothing on this earth that could compare to the embrace of my Lord. I was madly in love.

This apparently was not news for the crew at Restoration Ministries. The folks with whom I had been staying were joyous, untouched, but not surprised! This was an ongoing daily experience for deliverance ministers (exorcists) of the South. Just another day on the job!

*Hebrews 10:13: "For we know him that saith, vengeance belongeth to me, I will recompense saith the Lord."*

# I Gained Power

My entire healing had been imparted from one sister being led to say, "Jesus is alive." From one heart to another, under the instruction of God's perfect timing. I was finally developing some weapons. I was learning to stand, step out in faith and have victories in the spirit. All was well.

That day, I picked up the sword and kicked some evil butt, and it felt good. I had been pushed all the way back to death's door. My soul had been attacked. My entire body had been crippled by deception. I had almost been conned into giving up all of my foods again, going back to nothing!

Not this time. This time, I had gained power, not given power away! This was different; I was getting armed. I didn't have to live in torment anymore. I was no longer available for pain and oppression at the whims and wiles of evil.

*Psalm 23:5: "Thou preparest a table before me*
*in the presence of mine enemies: thou anointest*
*my head with oil; my cup runneth over."*

I had been attacked taking land, which is a very natural occurrence. I had stepped out in faith, and there was a counter-attack. A word battle is not meant to replace the faith of action. Action always has the loudest voice in the spiritual realm. Action is the word being demonstrated. It is good, however, to be prepared to have a sword in case of a post-victory attack.

*More action is also sufficient.* In other words: my point could have been made by simply busting the con by the action of faith and eating more food, a lot more food — the primal and power-ful retaliation of upping the ante.

# Chapter 23

## Glory to God in the Highest

I was accomplishing my purpose in coming to Green Cove, Florida. I was learning from God's "Holy Finest." I was very grateful to be able to get this very precious revelation from these authentic and experienced ministers of God. Sister Nellie, who was one of God's chosen at Restoration Ministries, always said to me, "Juliana, there are three important steps: surrender, step out in faith, and stand." I had just stood on my own.

## What God Was Teaching Me

I realized what Paul meant when he said, *"Brethren, I count not myself to have apprehended: but this one thing I do, forgetting those things which are behind, and reaching forth unto those things which are before, I press toward the mark for the prize of the high calling of God in Christ Jesus." (Philippians 3:14)*

I was getting an understanding of the importance of that revelation! Never look back! I was taught to take it to the top, cutting to the chase of God's ultimate authority over all things. His supreme will, and claiming His truth above all else, took precedence over anything else that I could possibly do.

> Deuteronomy 11:24: *"Every place whereon the soles of your feet shall tread shall be yours ..."*

## My Healing Was about Spiritual Empowerment

Up until this revelation and demonstration, I had believed that my healing was about my personal integrity. I had a belief that all illness came from disempowerment and giving power away. I thought that illness was from compromising integrity and submitting to idols. That is, of course—on some level—true, but truer still was the fact that I was redeemed from error.

*These compromises and idolatries were not my sins. They were attacks of my old nature; I was, in fact, two.* I was redeemed, translated by one blood offering to be the seed of God, my spiritual essence. My spiritual self could not sin; it was impossible. I was created in the image and likeness of God. (Genesis 1:27) *"Whosoever is born of God doth not commit sin; for his seed remaineth in him: and he cannot sin, because he is born of God." (1 John 3:9)*

## His Grace Is Sufficient
## (2 Corinthians 12:9)

I was not some poor, worthless victim, being punished by God; I was not some compromised soul on this earth. No, I was Holy, as He is Holy. His grace would be more than sufficient. Grace rules; enforcing His grace was the lesson that I had to learn. God's spiritual authority and grace have absolute dominion on this earth! No matter what the circumstance!

> *2 Corinthians 4:7: "But we have this treasure in earthen vessels, that the excellency of the power may be of God ... "*

## I Had Divine Rights

I had been given dominion and had rights here on earth! God-given rights. I could retaliate any blocks to God's grace. I could take back my health, my peace, food, clothes, etc. I was no longer a victim of spiritual foul play.

*Ephesians 1:21: "Far above all principality, and power,
and might, and dominion, and every name that is named,
not only in this world, but also in that which is to come."*

## The Battle Is for Identification

I had gotten sick by not knowing who I was in Christ and believing in the disempowering ways of the world. To add to that undermine, I was then conned into thinking I could fix myself. My only problem was that I was dealing with the wrong self. My own works would never heal me. No one, through correcting his or her character flaws, could expect healing.

Healing is separation, sanctification, a dividing asunder of soul and spirit. *Healing is simply opposing the impostor!*

*Hebrews 4:12: "For the word of God is quick, and powerful,
and sharper than any two-edged sword, piercing even to the
dividing asunder of soul and spirit, and of the joints and the
marrow, and is a discerner of the thoughts and intents of the heart."*

## Piggyback

I simply had to piggyback on a victory that was already established. For me, as a psychologist, this was not easy to grasp. It didn't matter if I were right or wrong, compromised, in integrity, a jerk, or a queen. What mattered was that I knew that I was healed by God and that His grace was sufficient! My sins, my mistakes, were forgiven by grace.

*John 1:7: "For the law was given by Moses,
but grace and truth came by Christ Jesus."*

## Appointed Time

I wanted to stay and be a part of this community. Rachel wanted me to stay. But we both knew that God had another plan; I was led to leave. I have found that the only real error in most situations was "staying too long at the fair." I had gained so much, but it was time for me to move on. I still had some chemical sensitivities and needed more healing. God was telling me to go home, that there were things I had to learn from God alone. I was finished with my victory in Florida. I had gotten what God wanted me to get.

## We Say Goodbye

The first person I said goodbye to was Pastor's wife Rachel. We had developed a relationship; we loved each other with the love of God! She shared her truth with me. "Juliana, two weeks ago I heard from God that it was time for you to go, and I didn't tell you because I wanted you to stay."

I shared mine. "I did the same thing, Rachel. I made believe I didn't hear! I know it's over."

We both laughed. We knew that if I stayed any longer "stuff" would begin to happen; we would be out of God's plan and his leading. We accepted that and knew that God's decision had foresight!

I continue to this day to see the timing aspect of God in everything that I do. It is above everything. It is spiritual law, the rule of the spirit. Grace is by faith. Faith will always be led by the spirit.

*Galatians 5:18: "But if ye be led of the Spirit,*
*ye are not under the law."*

## Stuff Happening

In other words, whatever our original problems were that created a disharmony, that interference (problem) is not what it appeared to be. The only true error was that you or I were not led by the spirit. *We were mislead. The impostor led us. That's all that really happened.* The grace of God covers all error.

Rachel drove me to the airport and we shared wonderful things of the Lord together. It was a glorious day of sisters edifying each other in our Lord! She shared some very special things that God had told her specifically to share. I promised her that I would not reveal any of the details. I will say this: I went home with clothes on my back, and I was actually overweight. I left with God's grace and much healing — with so much more in imparted wisdom and friendships, and a new family in God.

## Food: God's Cosmic Joke

Rachel lovingly dropped me off at the airport. I sat peacefully in the plane on my way back home. I had a radically different mentality from the one I had arrived with! I had decreased in my flesh and increased in my spirit.

*John 3:30: "He must increase, but I must decrease."*

## Counting Blessings

I had been supernaturally blessed by the greasiest pork, beef, French fries, and daily Dairy Queen ice cream. Southern-fried cooking not only didn't upset my stomach, I had overcome my digestive problems! I had overcome my allergic reactions! It clearly wasn't about the food.

The junk food was God's cosmic joke. If God were a Jewish mother, it would have sounded like this: "I told you so. Eat already." I weighed a hundred and thirty-two pounds—much more than I had ever weighed in my life!

God had His own ways of busting the con of deceptions.

*1 Corinthians 4:5: "Therefore judge nothing before the time until the Lord come, who both will bring to light the hidden things of darkness, and will make manifest the counsels of the hearts: and then shall every man have praise of God."*

# Chapter 24

## On My Own Again

I went home to my nontoxic Santa Barbara house. No land there — it was time to move on! I clearly heard from the Holy Spirit that it was not about my clinging to anyone else's ministry. God had a new purpose. I was being prepared for my next promotion! God had a plan, but it was about my moving on independently! I had to grow in God solo. I had to conquer these victimizations of the generational law with my own authority in Christ!

I was not without attacks after I returned home. I was, however, able to eat, wear clothes, and was much less chemically sensitive. I had achieved a major victory in Green Cove. I had retaliated against much deception. I was alive, eating, and hoped to go all the way with God. This path had power beyond my understanding. I was compelled to obey!

I was just beginning to see reality, to become my true nature. I knew that there was only one way to accomplish this. I got power by taking land, by stepping out in faith. That action of faith evoked God and His grace! It was about possessing the land, and I had much more land to take!

## Busting Another Con

One of my many medical diagnoses was an illness called "Chronic Fatigue Syndrome." I had lost much of my belief in these physical symptoms and now considered them to be lying symptoms of error.

The impostor of my soul would always like to present painful physical symptoms to undermine my newly gained authority. I was being challenged!

Evil knew that since I was now alone, this could become an opportunity to disempower me, an opportunity to take my newly gained understanding of faith. I had stepped into "retaliation faith," and my opposition was losing ground rapidly. Evil took a shot at my body.

## The Hostile Mentality of Chronic Fatigue

I enjoyed ten fairly high, healthy, faith-filled days upon my return from Green Cove. On the eleventh day, I awoke on my new, one hundred percent cotton futon (an upgrade of the glass table), and I was immobilized once again! I was de-energized, weakened; I felt exhaustion in every muscle in my body, every bone, and every limb. I could hardly move my physical body off of my new bed. I was so tired one would think I hadn't slept in a month. All I had been doing was sleeping. Still, I desired to sleep more.

## Tomorrow

Every day I woke up with worsening symptoms. I was becoming more fatigued. Each and every day, it became harder to get up! I was in a battle; I was cognizant of that. I was unable to activate my dominion. I had to take my will back from the impostor, to rise above it. Every day I felt worse, more drained, heavier, and more powerless. I was weakened by deception. I knew that's all it was—deception. I was convinced of that. I believed that with all my heart.

I rebutted half-heartedly, sans conviction. I was too tired to feel passion. I was an apathetic warrior! I attempted to engage deception in a passive dialogue. "Tomorrow," I said every day.

"Tomorrow I will get up and move on; tomorrow I will take the victory over your lie ... tomorrow ... I will take my life back ..."

This went on for eight days. Each day was more difficult; my body was heavier, my mind cloudier. Each "tomorrow," I was more exhausted than the day before. I was not gaining territory.

My old self was actually hyping me by consoling me with the illusion of a future "pie-in-the-sky liberty." I was being lulled into denial. The carnal nature was being very seductive in its demonic technique. The devil, after all, had a lot of experience in creating a vegetative state. What experienced warrior would allow this type of thought?

"Tomorrow. Tomorrow I will be who I am in Christ! I will sleep another twenty-four hours and then I will arise and be in my authority in Christ. Tomorrow I will awaken in righteousness (1 Corinthians 15:34) and bring my flesh under subjection ... Give me time."

I knew the truth but didn't have the strength to implement it. It was a position of conflict. I was a victim of oppression, although I knew it to be a lie! What a strange dichotomy. I had seen too much in Green Cove, Florida, to go back to that kind of bondage.

## The Decision

On the ninth day of this torture, I began to realize that I would have to stand! Literally. I would have to stand. Get up!

I would have to take this disease—this Chronic Fatigue impostor character—on! I made my decision. I would get up! Get out of bed!

"I've had it," I said, feeling more exhausted from my warfare not being acknowledged, not even being heard. I was hanging on ... It was, after all, a word war.

I would have to put a little faith in my words ... up the ante with a little action. Action required movement.

"You're not hearing me," I declared. "I am getting up, and when I get up, I am staying up. If I never lie down again, this is over! I will no longer submit to this deception. I will walk. I will run. I will not sit. I will not lie down. I have had it! I will not be conned into a rest position ever again. This is my life, and I am taking it back! This attack is over!"

This time, I meant it! My decision was made! I was getting up. "I am getting up," I continued. "I will stay up. I will not go back to this bed until this oppression is broken. If it does not end, then I will die standing, but I will not lie down!" My position was clarified.

## Identity Restored

My body, my carnal nature—now under my command—responded to the threat of my authority, knowing that it was authentic. Suddenly, and quite automatically, I arose. I was thrust up in spiritual power.

I had new power. My voice was now booming with a new depth, its volume increased! "I will not be controlled by chronic fatigue or any other lying physical symptom. You are a chronic deceiver. You are a chronic liar. I am not subject to your wiles; the power of Christ rests within me. I will not live as you," I declared. "I will not live lifeless."

This was the moment I had been waiting for: the moment when my regenerated spirit would rise up and do battle! In my true identity of righteousness, this Chronic Fatigue Syndrome was toast!

## The Amazing Thing

The minute my authentic threat was communicated, it all broke. All of my pain went away! It was gone; a powerful energy went through my body like a flash of light. The attack was broken. I had energy. I had power! I was radically and spiritually alive. I had spoken myself into my true nature, and my spirit knew what to do. I had taken my will back. I had overcome passivity. My weakened will had been strengthened by my ability to separate myself from the impostor.

My very choosing to disagree with the perceptions of evil had empowered my essence.

I stepped out of my bed effortlessly, with tremendous vibrancy, and went on with my day, my life. I have never had another symptom of the carnally contrived and illusionary "Epstein Barr Virus" or "Chronic Fatigue Syndrome."

I had stepped into resurrection power ... I was living the born again reality! The promise of dominion on this earth was mine to appropriate. My spirit could find its own way! I had an inner helper, the Holy Spirit. I could surrender to it, and the spirit of God would take over!

With that attack under subjection, I had to continue on in my purpose with God. I had returned to Santa Barbara to move on, to get out of my nontoxic asylum, my "safe" house. The opposition to my empowerment didn't like that. That was what the attack was really about — "chronic" procrastination of my inevitable mastery over evil. At that time, however, I still had some health problems to conquer.

## A Motivating Prayer

I was grateful to be eating, but I was still not totally free. I was grateful to be alive, but I was still stuck in an environmentally safe, nontoxic, chemical-free home. I went through a confusing time. I attended churches. I was prayed for. Nothing was really clicking, nothing was right. This went on for a season: getting prayed for, getting nowhere, until a concerned girlfriend was kind enough to bring her friend (a prayer warrior) to visit. He agreed to pray for my illness and chemical reactions.

He did just that. He went on and on, a very victimizing, undermining prayer. You know the kind of prayer — well meant, but it somehow makes you wrong. It was a prayer rooted in religious law and condemnation.

I did not want to be rude and insult my friends. Instead, I chose to war internally. While this lengthy prayer continued, I watched all words, all thoughts closely, separating myself from all erroneous identification … and then suddenly, there it was … God's word … God used me to deliver it! I was thrown up in the righteousness of the spirit and prophesied a word to my own heart. I began to speak the words of the spirit.

## God's Prophetic Word

*"I will not heal you or deliver you anymore, my daughter. If I do, you will always lose the healing. You will never hold onto anything. You will always be powerless. You, my daughter, will take the rest of your healing by faith, with your authority in Christ! Then no one, nothing, will ever be able to take anything away from you again."*

At first I was thrilled. I had finally heard from God again. The Almighty Himself had prophesied to me, for me, by me. I now knew what God wanted me to do … I would take the rest of my healing by faith, with my authority in Christ! I remembered what I was doing! I was learning my authority in Christ!

That was my personal way, my path. I had to appropriate my authority in Christ! I had given my power over to deception. I was powerless, that was my problem. It was not, however, my truth.

All power had been given unto me. Greater works would I do than even the Lord Himself. I was made in His Image and likeness. I was translated by one blood offering to be the right-eousness of God. I had His power, His dominion on this earth. I was not to be messed with or taken lightly. I had tremendous backup. Every place that my foot would tread would be mine! (John 14:12, Genesis 1:26, Hebrews 10:14)

153

The prayer warriors believed it was from their prayer that God had spoken. They also believed that we were all poor sinners, victims of life. They had not yet had the revelation of grace by faith.

They were praying in the old nature, which was exactly what God had delivered me from. I had to vehemently block the spirit of condemnation with every ounce of strength I had. Sin consciousness, condemnation and guilt had been instilled in these "warriors" via religion. They did not comprehend their true identity. And at that time, I was not grounded sufficiently in my newly regenerated spirit woman to enlighten them.

# Chapter 25

## The Con of Religion

Religion will seduce a person into listening to the voices of spiritless pastors, teachers, and self-appointed leaders. No breath in any of it. Hand-me-down words. Yesterday's manna. To have to repeat and rehearse "sermons" is not God's best. The Lord wants to deliver us from this repetition syndrome. *The Holy Spirit is not holding contrived, condemning services that focus on sin consciousness.*

Religion wants to deafen you to the voice of the Master. That's the con of religion. Religion wants you to think you can only get to God via another person, that you have no personal Kingdom. Religion wants you unaware of your position on earth. It doesn't want you to know that you are an independent contractor with God. You are not a codependent seeker of God through man. There can be nothing further from the truth.

## The Kingdom of God Is Within You! (Hebrews 12:28)

The purpose of this con is to keep you in your old nature, bowing to man, never knowing who you are. It is a spirit of control, mostly stemming from the manipulations of self-justification (a form of witchcraft), a front for the law.

I personally have never seen The Lord of Lords and King of Kings respond to whining, begging, and declarations of despair. Jesus loves you, the "you" He created. You are not the down-and-out "poor you" flesh. That is the enmity of God praying, pretending to be you.

155

*Romans 8:7: "The carnal mind is enmity against God."*

That type of prayer is a declaration of wrong identity. You might as well stand up and speak its lie directly. Say what it is really saying: "I didn't get it. I am still suffering in the flesh. There is no sanctification. He didn't do it. The Cross is null and void. Come back, Lord, and save me!"

*Romans 6:9: "Knowing that Christ being
raised from the dead dieth no more."*

The truth was that The Holy Spirit had been waiting to speak. I just needed to get my carnal mind, my thoughts and theirs, out of the way. I thanked my friend and the prayer warrior for the blessing and said goodnight ... I went to bed confident, ecstatic, and joyful! I had heard from God. That was all that was important. I was out of my wilderness. God was talking to me again! Hallelujah!

## Take What and How?

It took me a couple of days to come down from this "high," only to realize that I had no idea what God wanted me to do! I did not know how to proceed.

## His Thoughts Are Higher!

*Isaiah 55:9: "For as the heavens are higher than the earth, so are my
ways higher than your ways, and my thoughts than your thoughts."*

What authority in Christ? I needed a word to explain His word. What did God want me to do?

I knew that I had to move out of my safe house, but how? I was still chemically too sensitive for other homes. How was my authority in Christ (that I hadn't yet acquired) going to move me out of my nontoxic environment?

*Mark 1:22: "And they were astonished at his doctrine: for he taught them as one that had authority, and not as the scribes."*

## Nellie Inspires Me to Move

I became certain it was about my moving to a normal residence. I started looking for places to move into. I reacted to every house I saw! If the home had new carpet, I would have neck spasms, muscle pain, vomiting. Fresh paint would set off another series of reactions.

I focused all my daytime hours on looking for new places to live. Every home had its own series of complicated reactions. Some of the houses had recently been sprayed with pesticides, some with lawn weed killers. There were others that had detergent scents from laundry rooms, deodorizers, dog hairs, cat smells, cleaning fluids, dishwasher soaps, molds, dust. Life had toxins. I reacted to life!

I even reacted to the energy of neighbors too close by. I felt and reacted to everything. I looked at new rentals all day, every day, and then at night I would go home to the same old place. I was not getting anywhere. I couldn't find anything that I could live in. I couldn't find anything that I was able to walk into without having violent reactions! I remained in my safe house another day, another week, another month!

## Staying Too Long at the Fair

I had waited too long to move. I have noticed that God makes situations very undesirable when it's time to move on. I had to let go and move on. God was asking me to move into a new residence. I was in a dichotomy. I could not stay, and I could not go! I was reading the signs. They were clear. I needed some of that authority that God had mentioned! I was not accumulating any additional authority by staying in my "safe" home.

157

## You Will Get It by Removing Idols

I had already had the experience of forest fires breaking out when I tried to stay in an allegedly chemical-free home in Arizona. Every environmentally challenged person wants to move to clean air. It made perfect sense.

Whenever I would try the clean air move, I would have supernatural experiences of the ungodly kind. God's way of saying, "No, wrong direction. You won't get it here. You are adding idols. You will get it by removing idols."

Magnification of the negative is God's way of saying, "It is over! Let go; trust me. I can do better than this."

Idols are always available, and with them they bring the curse, which can be identified as strange and unnatural happenings, misfortune ... wrong time, wrong place ... the trap of the victimization of the law. A life of suffering.

## Backup

I called my old friends in Florida. I was two thousand miles away from any authentic spiritual support. There was a woman there, Sister Nellie, an integral part of the deliverance ministry.

Nellie was led to and was willing to stand with me on the phone. That was as good as it was going to get. I couldn't find anyone locally from Los Angeles to Santa Barbara who had the faith for my move into a normally toxic home.

Any time I would attempt to discuss it with a friend or any spiritually inclined person, I heard a lot of doubt. One minister actually said, "That's insane. What makes you think that will happen?"

I learned not to offer my faith ideas to folks without faith, not when it was about my personal stand.

> *John 10:27: "My sheep hear my voice,*
> *and I know them, and they follow me."*

## Sister Nellie

Nellie didn't have doubt. She was a perfect, sincere servant of God who had dedicated her entire life to the Lord. She was a woman of consistent and upright faith. She would not be moved.

As far as Nellie was concerned, if a person is having a physical reaction to something, the solution is to go towards it. She had no conflict. Jesus did it; you are healed by His Grace; appropriate it. Simply begin to walk towards God …

I called Nellie and told her my predicament. "Nellie, it is clear, I have to move on. I have faith for it. I believe it is God's will."

"I understand," Nellie said. "God is trying to root you out of there, to promote you."

"Yes, Nellie, but the strange thing is every time I go to see a potential rental, I get sicker. I can't walk in. I am so attacked. I walk through the house just to see it, and I go into physical pain. Nellie, sometimes it takes days to wear these symptoms down after I receive them!"

"It will change," Nellie said. "It will change once you move in."

"Nellie, if I leave this place and move, I cannot come back here. Where will I go? I will be homeless!"

## A Spirit of Procrastination

"It is a spirit of procrastination," Nellie concluded, "a spirit of procrastination keeping you stuck. Just go and pick a place."

"What should I look for?" I asked her.

"Take something you like, that's all you have to do. Take something you really like."

She continued in prayer. "We thank you, Father God, that you have not taken Juliana this far to not take her the rest of the way. She shall have her peaceful home. You shall provide it. We give you praise in advance for it.

"I speak to that spirit of procrastination in Jesus' name," she went on. "And I tell you, there is no power but the power of

God. You must cease and desist all your claims on Juliana's soul in Jesus's name. By the blood of the Lamb, you must go. Amen. "When you are attacked," Nellie said, "take communion."

> *1 Corinthians 10:16: "The cup of blessings, which we*
> *bless, is it not the communion the blood of Christ?"*

## Spiritual Facts

What was remarkable about Sister Nellie is that she would say things that were totally profound, but she said them in a very subtle way. When Sister Nellie spoke, there was absolutely no drama, no carnal emotions. She spoke very calmly, as if what she was saying was unimportant.

Nellie spoke in spiritual fact. She was not trying to impress anybody or look good. She was simply relating what she knew to be true. This made her very difficult to read; God had to reveal her to you. Once you understood her consecration to Christ, whatever she said you would do. You knew it was Jesus.

I asked Sister Nellie once if she had ever been married or had children. She replied, "No, but I have had many spiritual sons and daughters in the Lord."

Her appearance was the same as her personality: straightforward. She was tall, thin, hair pulled back, almost severe looking, with no makeup, fluff or frill, no "people pleasing" attire. As God revealed her to you, you saw her beauty. The sincerity of her heart shone through her "prudish" presentation. Deliverance ministry was not about personality or people, fame or reputation. You had to know beyond any shadow of a doubt that God was using someone on your behalf. I knew this about Nellie.

## Faith Was on the Way

Her prayer brought faith. She agreed with me; she sensed that it was time for me to move. I would pick a house I liked.

I had many questions, doubts, and a lot of pondering going on in my mind. What would happen if I couldn't live in the new house? How can I live in a house I couldn't walk into?

The spirit of procrastination wanted to distract me from further progress and was filling my carnal mind with questioning thoughts. What if? What then? Now what? More idols of the carnal mind. Fear and doubt! The impostor inquisition.

# Chapter 26

## Faith-Filled Inspiration

Nellie's interpretation of my situation was clear. The spirits of procrastination and fear were attacking me. I was immobilized. The only prerequisite for this house hunting expedition would be that I liked it!

"Take no concerns for your body," Nellie advised. "Move in and God will meet you there." Moving in was the key. God would meet me after the move; not on my plan, but on my demonstration, my action.

> Matthew 6:25: "Therefore I say unto you, take no thought for your life, what ye shall eat, or what ye shall drink ..."

Nellie was a faith-filled inspiration! She did not concern herself with worry if her prayers or words were anointed or not. The word was Jesus; it had its own strength. She had no hoopla tendencies; her faith was based on fact. When you spoke with Nellie, you were talking to a woman grounded on the Rock.

I was completely reassured of God's plan. It was clear in speaking with Nellie. I was being asked to step out in faith and God would meet me on the other side of that step. What else could possibly happen? My authority would be increased as needed! It would be increased by my step of faith. I would be enlarged! There was no other way!

I agreed with Nellie and took a house the very next day.

## Leaning Not on My Own Understanding
## (Proverbs 3:5)

I chose a place I couldn't walk into, and I moved in. It had a plethora of antagonists, but I liked it. It was a charming home in the Santa Barbara foothills. The house was like a little fairy tale cottage in a Hansel and Gretel setting. It was the perfect temporary rental.

I moved in by faith.

## I Shall Not Be Moved

Nellie believed that it was the Will of God, and I knew I had a stand partner who would not be tossed!

> Hebrews 12:28: "Wherefore we receiving a Kingdom
> which cannot be moved, let us have grace ..."

## Moving into a Real House

My "stand house" was selected rapidly. I chose to occupy it shortly thereafter. The home had two bedrooms, a living room, a kitchen, and dining room area. It was small, an older cottage, but lovely and quaint.

I report the rest now from an environmentally concerned perspective.

The first thing that I noticed when I walked into the home was the living room carpet, which was old and moldy. I could smell the dust and mold. The minute I walked into the house, my neck would go into my mold spasms! This also created pain in my shoulders and tightness in all my muscles, triggering a series of reactions, including a migraine. There was nothing I could do but wait it out. I had moved in.

The rental home was furnished. I had no furniture, so moving in was uneventful: a few plain brown paper bags full of clothing, a few plates, some kitchen utensils. I had not accumulated much in my last residence. All I had was God's promise of my future.

I avoided the living room; it was too intense. I would take that on later as I gained strength. I quickly passed through to a smaller room down the hall. This small back bedroom area faced the garden. It had a little sliding glass door and a patio. Simply adorable!

I allowed myself to feel the beauty for a brief moment, then it was right back to my dilemma. I had to choose a room to sleep in, a room that would become my stand room. I was allergic to everything in the home without exception. I would have to occupy this home room by room.

*Luke 19:13: "Occupy till I come."*

## The Back Bedroom

I moved into the back bedroom only because it was, in my estimation, less toxic than the front bedroom. I peeped into the front bedroom, got a sniff of a combination of things so vile I choked, shuddered, became totally confused and slammed the door shut. It was just too much for today. First day on the job!

The back bedroom, I thought, had a sliding glass door that provided a little air, an escape! I could never sleep outside, as some environmentally challenged folks do. That would be worse for me: the mold, the fumes, and the airborne allergens. It was not an option.

## A Toxic Paradise of Pressed Wood

There were enough intoxicants in this room to conjure up more than a little anxiety. The room was paneled with pressed wood. Pressed wood! I was well informed about pressed wood.

The entire environmentally sensitive community and its immune system specialists had pontificated on the subject at length.

Toxicologists were always quick to warn about the deadly poisons involved in the making of particleboard! Pressed wood was composed of imitation wood — shaved pieces of cardboard glued together. The it-can-kill-you-if-you-sniff-it toxic type of glue! The poisons of pressed wood glue could destroy your brain! I had heard that these particle and pressed wood boards can give off toxic fumes years after they had been constructed, even decades.

These pieces of particleboard were not nailed to the walls like real wood. They were glued on with more glue! All four walls were covered with the pressed-wood-paneled look — very attractive, very confrontational, and very deadly!

It is best to be naive in these areas of research.

> *1 Corinthians 2:5: "That your faith should stand not in the wisdom of men, but in the power of God."*

## Gas Heat

The room had a gas heater attached to the wall, right on top of the glued pressed wood. More fumes! It became apparent that my landlords had not considered the fact that the heat would release poisonous glue fumes in the pressed wood.

*They did not sleep in this room. That's probably why they're still alive*, self-exaltation remarked in my thoughts.

## I Turn on the Gas (A Step into Proper Identity)

I took a step of faith and put the heat on. *I'm here*, I thought, *I have to go for it. I am certainly in the trust-God-or-die category now! I might as well go all the way.*

*Gas heat*, my carnal mind acknowledged. *You're sleeping in a room with gas heat?*

I already had more power than I had in my safe house. I was able to discern my thoughts! A perk of faith! One step of faith and I was already being made separate from the voice of the old nature.

"Are you sure?" evil questioned. "Why not use your portable electric heater? This is not about asphyxiation; it is about moving on, having a comfortable home, going on with your life. Be gentle with yourself," the spirit of self-exaltation continued, "you've been through enough!"

## I Occupy

I chose to carry all of my possessions into this little room. It was here I would begin my stand. I was utterly alone. All I had in the entire world was with me. I would either gain from here or have this be what I would leave the earth with.

## A Final Attempt to Change God's Plan

The opposition continued its banter. It was trying to play the "alone" card. "Don't put your bag near that gas heater. If you have to run out of this house, you do not want all your possessions to be toxic. Your clothes will be ruined. Everything will be destroyed by the smell of gas!

"What if the gas kills you in the night, poisons you to death?" the imposter went on. "No one knows that you are here. There is no one to check up on you; you are totally alone in this world. No family, no friends. This is not a good idea. You have no Plan B! You have nothing to fall back on in case of an emergency. No one knows where you are. No one will find you to revive you."

Sin consciousness was trying to hit me emotionally, to change my mind through the thoughts of the carnal mind — steal my hope, get me in self-pity, bring me down, and distract me from my potential victory. My opposition wanted to steal my stand.

The manipulation was too obvious. I was not that vulnerable to the "no one will find me" routine. I had more important things on my mind! I remained conscious. My step of faith had given me the power of sanctification. I was able to draw the line.

"This stand is between me and God. What I have is enough for God! God will work with it. He will meet me where I am," I replied.

> Psalm 62:5: "My soul, wait thou only upon
> God; for my expectation is from Him."

## Stakes Are High

I was not feeling the loneliness, somehow. I was actually feeling quite hopeful. I was expecting a miracle! Who I really was—a quickened spirit in my right identity—had a sense of being led by God. The human seed had its own fears and pre-disposed evaluations ... I was feeling hopeful, not certain.

I lay down on the bed that was in the furnished room — a real bed, not a 100% cotton futon, not a glass table, not an old army cot. A normal bed, with normal bedding. I put my head on a real pillow, a comfortable and normal headrest. *Am I dreaming? A real pillow?*

*What's the difference?* I thought. *With the gas heat on, a few bedding fumes of foam and synthetic materials will get lost in the shuffle, eaten up by larger toxins.* I was not warring for a bed here. The stakes were higher than bedding! This was life or death. God would deliver me or not. He would show up or not. I would wake up healed or I would have nowhere to go, no place to turn. This was it!

I got up one more time to shut my sliding glass door. It was getting cooler; it was nighttime in Santa Barbara. I returned to my bed. Lying there, eyes wide open, I found myself smelling and listening to the noises of the gas heat going on, going off.

## As Toxic As It Gets

The old nature (the flesh) was not in agreement with my new surroundings and it took this opportunity to summarize its position. "Oh my God, oh my God. The sliding door is closed. The windows are closed. There is no air in here, none that can be breathed by even normal, healthy people. You are in a regular bed, fumes are exuding from the walls and the gas heater. All in this tiny room. Can't you smell this room? Can't you smell what is going on in here?"

The impostor was hysterical! "Where is your nose? This is toxic! Toxic! As toxic as it gets! Have you gone mad? This is not a stand; this is suicide! You're in denial. You are in total denial!"

## I Am Here, Lord

I put my eyes back on Jesus. "Here I am, Lord, in a perfectly charming bedroom, the quintessential rustic Santa Barbara cottage-style cabin, with a lovely sliding glass door that opens out to a charming garden, facing the extraordinary Santa Barbara mountains. Breathtaking! Here I am, Lord. I am here. I put my trust in you."

The enmity was still influencing my take. "This could go either way," deception sneered. I ignored the comment. In faith, in victory, this was ideal. I loved the cottage. This could be heaven or death row.

My regenerated spirit had its own opinion. *This is great; this is the beginning of my real life.* I fell asleep, lulled by the sound of a gas heater producing fumes.

# Chapter 27

## The Next Day

When I awoke the next morning, the very second my eyes opened, the carnal mind started talking fast and aggressively. "Look at you. Look at you," it declared, premeditated entanglement pouring out of its evil consciousness, venom more disabling than any gas heater. "You can't move," deception went on. "You're immobilized; you might be paralyzed, asphyxiated. Smell this room. Open a window, throw all the windows and doors open immediately! Get out of here! Get out!"

## Drunk in Fumes

I—"me"—could not think. My true mind would not work; my thoughts would not form. I was incoherent.

"You're not incoherent," the aggression continued. "You're drunk in fumes. This is what it feels like to be poisoned! This is what it feels like when you have environmental illness and sleep in a toxic room! You have finished yourself off. You will never recover from this self-inflicted exposure!"

## I Push Myself

I pushed myself off the side of my new bed with all my strength. The enmity of God was not finished speaking. "You cannot move; you're exhausted. You're on the floor. That is not getting up out of bed; that is rolling onto a floor. You're going to die in this house!"

I had to pull out of this somehow. I had to muster up the courage to call Nellie.

I was unable to see; my eyes were swollen shut. I crawled to the bathroom. I was hanging on. I grabbed the bathroom towel rack to hold myself up. I glanced at myself through eye slits. I looked green and swollen, like a boxer who had just lost a fight. I pushed my back up against the wall while more hostile suggestions were attacking me.

"This is all from the fumes you breathed in all night long. They have taken their toll. What did you expect? You have environmental illness! You have slept in a room with pressed wood, gas, synthetics, and no air. You are sicker now than you have ever been in your life. Living in the street would be better than this. You cannot live here! You didn't make it! God is not in this. God did not deliver you, not this time. Get out now! Save yourself while you have some life left."

## Where Is God?

I was heavy—drugged, I believed, from toxins. I had no focus, none. I could hardly breathe. I was gasping for air.

*What can I do?* I wondered. *Where is God?* I pushed myself up using the towel rack as a lunge point, a booster. I pushed and shimmied from one wall to another. I still did not have the strength to walk. I tried to walk on my own and my legs gave way. I grabbed onto the bathroom door handle. I was then between two rooms, the living room and bathroom.

*If I can get to the living room,* I thought, *I can get to the phone and call Nellie.* I gave myself a mission. I would drag myself, shoulder-to-shoulder, using the walls to hold me up — one small side step at a time to the table in the dining room area, where the phone was. My body was lifeless; it was like dragging dead weight.

I didn't feel like talking to anyone. I wasn't bubbling with the desire to communicate. I just wanted to tell Nellie what was happening. Just a contact: "Hello. I'm dying. Bye!"

I didn't know what I would say. Maybe Nellie wouldn't even be home. It seemed like an hour of effort to get across the walls. Everything hurt. I had no flexibility; I was as heavy and stiff as wood. Perhaps I had merged with the pressed wood!

## I Had a God Problem

I finally got to the chair and collapsed on it as I tried to gather my thoughts. What was my problem again? Oh right, my problem was definitely "Where was God?" I had a "where was God" problem. That was my conclusion: if God were here, I would not have this problem.

The minute I took some mental control and described my problem, the impostor chimed in. "Yeah, where is God? Where is God now? This is a little past the eleventh hour. This looks like a big no-show to me!"

I picked up the phone. I couldn't see the numbers on the dial; my eyes were still too swollen. I dialed "0" and the operator directed me to Information, where the person gave me Nellie's number. But each time I got it, I would forget it. There were no pens or paper on the table to write it down. I would get the number, forget it, and go through the whole process again until finally, on the fourth try, I remembered it. I then got an operator to connect me. My brain was barely functioning.

## Nellie Was Home

"Hello."

"Nellie, you're home!"

"Who is this?" Nellie asked. She didn't recognize my voice.

"It's me, Juliana," I said. "It's me. I slept in the house in the back bedroom with the gas heat on. I am in the land, but God

**171**

didn't heal me! I'm so sick. I am unable to think clearly. Nellie, I think I am poisoned."

"Pray with me," Nellie said.

"I can't, Nellie." I was unable to think. "I can't feel."

"Pray in the spirit then," Nellie said.

"Nellie, you're not getting this. I am not going to make it. I can't live here and I can't go back. I have never been sicker! Where is God?"

> *Psalm 46:5: "God is in the midst of her; she shall not be moved: God shall help her, and that right early."*

Nellie picked up the Bible, undaunted, and felt led to read Psalm 1. She began to read out loud, calmly, as if nothing were wrong.

*I am dying; she is not tossed. I am freaking out; she is not disturbed, not upset in the least.* Her faith had not been touched. God had chosen well. I may only have had only one person to help me, but the one I had could not be moved by evil. She was worth an army of unrighteous folks. One good, faithful servant.

Nellie was continuing to read Psalm 1 from the Bible, something about my receiving ungodly council. "You are receiving ungodly council," she declared.

No one would dispute that. She read it again. We were both feeling it now. There was a power in the words she had been led to read.

She was not just a Bible reader in a religious fashion. That was not what was going on. Sister Nellie was reading His light-filled word, knowing its power, in full faith and knowledge in the word's ability to deliver me on its own merit. She knew that Jesus Christ would back His word.

> *1 Peter 1:25: "But the word of the Lord endureth for ever."*

## The Entrance of Thy Word Giveth Light
## (Psalm 119:130)

That entire week, I kept seeing and hearing the same scripture, in my own studies and everywhere I went: "The entrance of thy word giveth light." That one scripture seemed to appear everywhere. I had never noticed that scripture before, and suddenly I was inundated with it. Nellie, who is not easily discouraged when it comes to the Lord, was very aware of the substance of that fact: "the entrance of His word giveth light." I had heard her comment on that verse in the past.

But then, in that moment, I was hardly hearing her Bible reading. I was in such despair. I had just lost my perfect oasis. I was utterly disenchanted. I was on a stand not being met by God; I had nowhere to go from there. The life I had hoped for was over.

Nellie continued to read Psalm 1. No prayer, nothing else, just Psalm 1, very calmly.

## Ungodly Council Continues

The mind of my soul, the impostor of my spiritual identity, was evaluating the situation with a slew of opportune, hostile suggestions. "You are homeless and dying, soon to be out in the street with fumes, toxic air and molds where you cannot survive. You have just slept in a toxic room—in the worst room you have ever slept in your life, a room that had enough disgusting toxins to kill ten environmentally ill people. You are sick, nauseous, ugly, swollen beyond recognition, and you are getting biblical news, ungodly council. You can't live in this house," self-exaltation babbled. "That is your reality!"

The generational carnal mind went on a rampage! "You're dying, that's all. It's over. You will not live another day. This was the dumbest, most psychotic thing you have ever done in your

173

entire life, turning that gas heat on! Everyone was right. This is not a way to be healed; this is a way to be exterminated!"

I was being inundated with bad news, condemned and accused of being misled, of being ill advised.

Nellie was still reading Psalm 1, *"… Blessed is the man that walketh not in the counsel of the ungodly, nor standeth in the way of sinners, nor sitteth in the seat of the scornful. But his delight is in the law of the Lord; and in his law doth he meditate day and night. And he shall be like a tree planted by the rivers of water, that bringeth forth his fruit in his season; his leaf also shall not wither; and whatsoever he doeth shall prosper. The ungodly are not so: but are like the chaff which the wind driveth away.*

*"Therefore the ungodly shall not stand in the judgment, nor sinners in the congregation of the righteous. For the Lord knoweth the way of the righteous …"*

## Nellie Reads On

Nellie was reading on, undaunted. I was still sitting in a dazed state at the table in the dining area. The table faced the front door. There was a hallway between the living room and the front door. I was actually positioned in a straight line, about thirty feet from the front door.

Suddenly, my eyes were drawn to the door, where something grabbed my attention. I thought that someone was at my door. "Oh no," my carnal mind evaluated. "That's all I need now, a visitor! I have to hide. I will be very quiet, and no one will know I am here. I cannot handle anything else right now!"

I disconnected from Nellie and her Bible reading. My concern was this new situation at my front door. I did not hear anyone on the premises; there was no bell ringing, no knocking, but something or someone was out there. I could feel it, sense it!

I focused on the door. At first, what I was seeing looked like a large glare from the sun. A big sunspot! But it was more than a sunspot. I knew that intuitively. A sunspot does not have a presence; it is not a being. This was *alive*. I could feel an energy! I kept a close watch; I was drawn to the door, compelled to observe. I did not want any interference right now. I needed deliverance, escape, peace, not intrusion.

Then the sunspot started to enlarge. At first it was on the other side of my door, on the outside. The light around the oversized spot was bright enough that it could be perceived right through a thick wood door! It was as if my door had become transparent! I watched as my door became encapsulated in light. This light was trying to get into my house! It wanted to enter; it had my full attention as it succeeded in pushing its way through my front door, till the bright light was inside my home! I was mesmerized. I could see nothing else. Next, the "light" consumed the hallway. It happened so fast that I was unable to report it to Nellie. I just sat there stunned as this embodiment of brilliant light moved through my house!

Ambulatory illumination silently meandered through the hall. It went through the hall and then into my living room as if it were looking for something. It had a determination about it. It was there on business. It appeared to have a mission, a direction.

I was shocked, not fearful. It happened so fast that I didn't have time to interpret what could be going on. I continued to observe as this incredible force of radiant light started to focus on a more direct path. It then headed straight towards me. It looked like I would be the target. Then, the light found me and stopped in its tracks. It stood directly in front of me for a moment ... stood there and paused ... and in that moment I realized that this was the light of God! This was the light of the Lord Jesus Christ Himself!

> John 8:12: "Then spake Jesus again unto them, saying, I am the light of the world: he that followeth me shall not walk in darkness, but shall have the light of life."

**175**

# A Light Injection

As soon as I had that realization, the light entered my body. This huge embodiment of spiritual illumination went through my body. I was speechless. I felt the heat, the fire of God, literally, as it went into my solar plexus area and out the other side. The light did not linger or go into different body parts. It just went through me, as if I were getting a giant injection of the Light of the Lord. Then it was gone.

Nothing else happened. Just a light visit. No revelation, no conversation, no commands. The light of God went in, went out, and all my symptoms were taken with it — all my pain, all my oppression, my mental attack, my lupus, and my environmental illness. Ungodly council had been silenced! I was no longer swollen. I was beautiful; I could feel it. I was free!

The entrance of His word had brought light to my home, through my door, through my body, and delivered me! All I had as a witness was Sister Nellie, two thousand miles away — one woman, a senior citizen, on the telephone, a veteran in the Lord. She was my God line. Nellie had remained not only sane, which is a good thing when you are being mentally tormented, but also very grounded, and absolutely centered in Christ.

*Isaiah 55:11: "So shall my word be that goeth forth out of my mouth: it shall not return unto me void, but it shall accomplish that which I please, and it shall prosper in the thing whereto I sent it."*

# Chapter 28

## I Feel the Presence of the Lord

Nelly felt it over the phone. She was hanging on the line, praying and still reading Psalm 1. I wasn't aware of her for a few minutes. I was in another dimension; the dispensation of grace had overcome my flesh!

"Nellie, I was being healed," I said.

"I know," she responded. "Jesus Christ just walked into your house, didn't He? I felt the presence of the Lord."

*Psalm 16:11: "… In thy presence is fullness of joy …"*

## We Rejoice

We were laughing now, praying, thanking, worshipping—having a grand time in the Lord. Incredibly, all of my symptoms had miraculously disappeared as this light permeated my body. I felt great. Could this be true? Here I was in a toxic house, and I was feeling great!

Nellie suggested that I go out and eat more junk food to celebrate this victory. She thought that I should celebrate by going out and eating pancakes and ice cream. I agreed but didn't go quite that far. I ate my normal meal. I was happy.

*Whew! I can live in a house! I can live.* I was so grateful to God. Imagine God walking through my door with His awesome light and walking right through my body, to deliver me. It was unimaginable.

*The word of God did not return void; that word of God for me
was alive and active, sharper than any two-edged sword. It had
penetrated to divide soul and spirit, joints and marrow; it
judged the thoughts and intents of my heart. (Hebrews 4s:12)*

## High in God

I was high in the Lord! I had been dead, and now I had life,
clothes, a home to live in, and a bed to sleep in. I could eat
food. I had new hope and excitement about living. I consecrated
myself to Jesus and prayed. "I have a predestined purpose to
serve you, Lord. I love you, and I am very, very grateful. You are
everything to me, you are all I have, all I need, all I desire!"

I had no intention of letting go of the hem of His garment.

*Matthew 14:36: "As many as touched were made perfectly whole."*

## Going from Stand to Stand

*Zechariah 13:9: "And I will bring the third part through
the fire, and will refine them as silver is refined ..."*

I was then able to live in the new rental house, and I was
once again learning to stand. I had learned again that I couldn't
evaluate something from the other side of the mountain. I had to
walk into my territory via faith and confront the giants in the
land. There was no other way I could be healed. Nothing else
had worked after years of trying.

## Faith as Healer

God's plan of taking it by faith was healing me. It was
becoming an extraordinary journey. Everything was becoming a
stand. I was going from stand to stand!

My miracle would never have happened in my environmentally safe house. I would be the same me, have the same problems, same God, same faith, same parents, same path, same
body, same destiny ... but my health would have continued to

worsen in an environmentally safe house, because there was no faith in it.

I was learning that no faith equals no grace; grace is by faith. (Ephesians 2:8) Faith is in the action of demonstrating that God is in control. It was too far-fetched for my thinking. It was an unknown concept to me at this time, this faith-as-healer thing. I had been blessed. I had the privilege of tapping into the power of God ... retaliating, and I was just beginning!

*2 Corinthians 3:18: "But we all, with open face beholding as in a glass the glory of the Lord, are changed into the same image from glory to glory, even as by the Spirit of the Lord."*

## Taking More Land

There was nothing I could do but take more land, and there was much land to be taken. I would not be running out of land for a very long time. I still haven't. There's always land. There is the ongoing land of sanctification. There is the land of the spirit, living more of your true nature. There is the land of dominion. All of this is available to you by faith.

*1 Corinthians 3:18: "If any man seemeth to be wise in this world, let him become a fool, that he may be wise."*

I have noticed that there are two types of people when it comes to land: one is humble and wants to be promoted in the Lord, and the other is in denial. Denial sounds like this: "God is blessing me; it's all good!" Or the religious take: "Be careful; you don't want to tempt God"—as if faith is an affront to God. These are really statements of doubt in God's grace.

The land of denial has to be conquered before any real move of God can be demonstrated. There is no light in denial! It does not make a believer unblessed to need to step out and take land. Land is a way of deepening our relationship with God.

There is no faith in denial! It is a control move of the impostor! The impostor wants you to avoid any empowerment and authority over it! If you have not taken any land, your flesh (the thoughts of the carnal mind) might be running your life.

*Matthew 6:33: "But seek ye first the Kingdom of God, and His righteousness; and all these things shall be added unto you."*

## Mold Land
## (The Moldy Bedroom)

There were other rooms in my rental house that I could not walk into. There was one room that was so full of dust and mold that no one wanted to walk into it. I knew that if I had come this far I would have to continue and take back all the things I had given up in my illness. I decided to sleep in that room. What was the difference, really? I was either in authority over my body or I was not. I had dominion or I did not. Dominion was not selective; it was inclusive of all things.

*Psalm 8:6: "Thou madest him to have dominion over the works of thy hands; thou hadst put all things under his feet."*

I ignored the dust, the mold smells, and the comments of others who had seen the room. I moved into it. I had newfound confidence. I knew what God wanted me to do: stand alone. There was no Nellie in the wings. I was to learn and grow in the spirit. I had the zeal of a newly healed woman.

## Night One

The first night that I slept in the new bedroom, I was confident that I would be delivered immediately the next morning. My expectations were high. I had no reason not to expect total and immediate grace; God had met me every step of the way. There had been no delays, not since I had first started retaliating and taking back my land, not since God had started teaching me faith.

*Romans 6:14: "For sin shall have no more dominion over you: for ye are not under the law, but under grace."*

## Morning One

An immediate deliverance wasn't what happened. When I woke up, I didn't feel well at all. I wasn't that concerned about my body and mood; I knew that I would wear down the lying symptoms as the day progressed. I certainly wasn't going to give the room up. I would sleep in that room again that night. I went on with my day, pushing through it half alive.

## Night Two

After sleeping in the new bedroom on the second night, I felt worse. I was confident that I would be delivered, that these reactions would be worn down. I would not be seduced by the deceptions. I knew by then the lies that could be created by the carnal mind and the symptoms that would accompany deceitful suggestions! The mind was the body. Thoughts created the body's sensations, whether pain or joy. The problem was: there were thoughts I couldn't see, lies I couldn't defend. I had to get a little higher in the Lord to perceive the schemes of evil.

## Night Three

I slept in the unsafe bedroom again. I was starting to feel very toxic. I couldn't imagine what was going wrong. I was standing, and yet, I wasn't being healed. I couldn't understand how that was possible. I went on with my day.

## Night Four

After sleeping in the room the fourth night, I began to become quite ill. I was starting to lose some of the foods that I had gained. I was having trouble urinating; my urine was becoming cloudy, and there was some blood in it. The opposition had intimidated me. I was staying in this room, but I wasn't winning the battle. I was stuck again.

Spirits of doubt and unbelief were badgering me. "This is unhealthy," doubt remarked. "You are losing foods. You are alive now because you can eat food again. Remember where you were when you were starving? Sixty pounds is not a joke. When you cannot eat, your whole body collapses. You of all people should know that. You have made tremendous gains. Why sleep in a disgusting, moldy room? There just is no reason to sleep in a room that makes you sick! No human being on this earth would sleep in a room that is toxic to them if they had a choice. You have a choice! What are you waiting for? You already have a kidney infection. You can hardly eat. Are you waiting to have no foods left? To be back where you were?"

There was a barrage of negativity aimed at undermining me. If I received it, my identity would be compromised! Evil was preparing its case, making its opening arguments.

## I Could Not Go Back

I was stalemated. I couldn't leave that room and return to the room that I was already delivered from because then I wouldn't be taking my land. If I returned to the other rooms, I would be backing down. I knew by then that if I allowed myself to be backed down, I would be available for defeat. I would jeopardize what I had already taken. I would be warring backwards, fighting old battles over and over again ... not advancing.

## Holding Fast

If I went back into the other bedroom, I would be retreating. I would not have the victory of the new room. I considered that move more dangerous than losing my foods. Here in the moldy room, I was at least in my land. I had a spiritual purpose; there, I would be relinquishing land.

I chose to stay in the unsafe moldy room, in which I was attacked. I had lost a few battles, but I was not out of the ballgame. I was not used to warfare defeat. I had become accustomed to walking in miracles.

## Lord, Lord, Lord!

Every day I sought the Lord. I was praying, seeking, asking, "What can I do? Lord, what do you want me to do? I came into this room by faith, and I'm not getting the healing I expected! Lord, what would you have me do? Where shall I sleep? What room is your will? Why am I not being met if I am in faith?"

That was what I couldn't understand. How was it possible that God was not meeting me? I knew it was God's will for me to take this room, to overcome all my reactions to this house. "What am I not seeing, Lord? What's so different about this room?"

The opposition had answers, had resolutions to all my questions. "Better move back to the old room," the devil commented. "It was peaceful, you were doing so well—best you've done in a long time. You were happy. Now you are sick and miserable. You'd better call a doctor about that kidney infection and get a professional opinion of your condition."

## No More Doctors

"I am not going to doctors," I retorted. That one I wasn't buying. I had seen too much, gone too far with God, to get conned into doctor calling. If I were sure of anything, it was the fruitlessness of that venture. I could tell myself to get out of a room. I didn't need medical help.

"You're right," the devil continued. "The doctors couldn't help you when you were dying. Why would they be able to help you if you get sick again? You had better get out of that room!"

## Where Are You, Lord?

"Do you want me to stay in this room or get out?" I asked. "What do you want me to do? I've done all I can, Lord. I am standing in my land waiting for you. Where are you?"

> *Ephesians 6:13: "Wherefore take unto you the whole armour of God, that ye may be able to withstand in the evil day, and having done all, to stand."*

## Go Back

My condition worsened every day. I didn't give up the room, but I was not getting better. I was losing foods daily. I was being mentally threatened. Every day in my thoughts I would hear, *You will lose all of your foods. You won't be able to eat. Get out of this room. It's not worth it! You are destroying your kidneys. Hasn't it been hard enough? Go back; enjoy this time. You can still eat some foods. You can still sleep and live in this house. Why ruin what you have? You deserve some peace. Take care of yourself. Go back. Retreat.*

It seemed the weaker I became, the more varied and aggressive the story got about my retreating to old territory.

## Spiritual Terrorism

I have found that the voice of evil will always threaten you in an attempt to make you lose the little bit of land that you have accumulated. It's a ploy to create a fear of losing what you have already gained. The impostor wants you so focused on holding on to what you have to keep you from moving ahead. It wants to make sure you are not accumulating any additional power over it. The voice of evil wants to push you back … arrest your progress … steal your victory. It suggests peace, peace, and there is no peace.

> *Jeremiah 6:14: "Peace, peace; when there is no peace."*

> *John 10:10: "The thief cometh not, but for to steal, and to kill, and to destroy: I am come that they might have life, and that they might have it more abundantly."*

## Day Eight

By the eighth day, things did not look good for me at all. I was now mostly just praying in that room, asking the Lord to lead me. My life was on hold. I was too sick to leave the house. Finally, I heard from God! I got my response. The King of Kings and Lord of Lords, the great I Am, the Holy Lord of Israel spoke to me. This is exactly what he said, no more, no less—just this command: *"Don't hold back on me now."*

*"Don't hold back on me now"* was my word from the Lord! I didn't get it. I thought, *This is really crazy! I'm in the room. I did not retreat! I can't eat. My kidneys are infected. How am I holding back?*

*"Don't hold back."* I believed that I had stepped out in great faith, and yet God was evaluating my position as someone who was holding back! I needed to know what I could possibly be holding back. I thought that this step of faith, my willingness to take this room, was enormous.

## "Don't Hold Back"

I began pondering this "don't hold back" concept. "Don't hold back; that makes no sense, Lord. What do you mean, *don't hold back?* Is this true? Am I holding back? *"Don't hold back."* What does that mean, *"don't hold back"*? Lord, I am not going back to the old bedroom! I have not given up this room! I will not give this room up!"

I heard nothing more, not one more word. God would say no more. El Shaddai had spoken, that was it. He had imparted what He wanted to say. He had given His revelation to His daughter: "Don't hold back."

Three little words: "Don't hold back." I have noticed that God is not a babbler; he is a God of few words. People who go on and on with these big, long, windy "thus sayeth the Lord" speeches are mostly entertaining their imaginations. God doesn't speak like Shakespeare; he created Shakespeare for that. God is God: profound, succinct, very plain, simple. Too simple for me, a complex human.

> *1 Corinthians 1:27: "But God hath chosen the foolish things of the world to confound the wise."*

> *1 Corinthians 3:19: "For the wisdom of this world is foolishness with God."*

*"Don't hold back."* I had to begin to agree with God, to start to see it his way. He was trying to tell me something. I was grateful to hear it. It had been a long nine days.

*"Don't hold back!"* Somehow I had to get in agreement with what I knew to be God's imparted word. "Yes, Lord, don't hold back. Yes, Lord, you are right. I praise you, Lord, for your word, for the revelation. I agree with you, Lord. I do not want to be someone who holds back. I want to give you my all! If I am holding something back, Lord, I want to release it! I will not hold back, I will not … I refuse to hold anything back."

And there it was … I had it. I was seeing it, feeling it. I felt the Holy Spirit pass the revelation into my heart! I knew it now. I knew that I had it. I understood what it meant! *"Don't hold back."* I received the meaning of God's directive word.

## Take What's Taking You!

I was being threatened about losing my foods; that I would not gain new foods as I had anticipated, and I would lose what I had already gained. When I saw it that way, it was very clear. His thoughts were higher ... a whole different line of thinking there. (Isaiah 55:9)

What I had to do, and what I had to understand, in God's eyes, is that what was being held back was where the faith attack actually was, not where I thought it was. I had to take that land, the land that was taking me, and take more of that specific land. I had to add a little land, up the ante a little bit. The stakes were high. I had more power than I could see; God was empowering my faith, enlarging my heart.

## What Was I Holding Back?

My eating was being threatened. *"You will not eat; you will lose the foods you have gained"* was the intimidation I had been listening to.

That was what was being held back. I had to retaliate. I had to go further. I was taking a beating being backed up. I was fighting the battle on the territory that my opposition had chosen. God was showing me spiritual strategy. *"You stepped out in faith, that was good. You stood, that is good. Now don't hold back. Don't give in, don't allow yourself to be threatened and bow down to lying symptoms. Hear what the Spirit is saying. End this attack."*

Move ahead of deception, up the ante, call the bluff ... retaliate ... and bust the con! Yes, I saw it. I had been blinded by the symptoms, tossed into fear. I either had faith or I didn't. I was healed or I was not. This was not a gray area. A gray area stand was penetrable! I was going to have to put my money down, so to speak (in this case, my body).

## Call the Bluff

In a card game, this would be called "calling a bluff." I was being told to call the bluff of the devil. It went something like this: "Impostor, let me see your hand! *I call you!* You have toxicity, kidney problems, and a threat of losing more foods. I have Jesus, His blood and grace. You think you can raise me on that? I know I am healed. I have faith to call your bluff, and I command you to show your real hand! I bust your con. I am on to you."

*Romans 13:1: "For there is no power but of God."*

I went out and ate those pancakes and ice cream, the foods that my Sister Nellie had prophetically and wisely suggested a few stands ago. I would not hold any foods back; I would not be threatened by doubt. I ate every food that I had not yet eaten, not yet taken back by faith till that moment. God had to have all power over food in my life. I took my power back from food again. I had to take all my food back once and for all — an eat-by-faith feast!

## I Saw It as God Saw It

I had the vision. I was beginning to see it as God saw it. With God's truth, I would eat all the foods I had not been able to eat before, foods that I would not have considered eating before I got into the conflict of the room. By the time I was finished pigging out, the threat was over. I felt great; my kidneys felt fine; my urine was clear. I had the joy and peace of a good victory. I had conquered the attack!

That night, I went back into that room and slept soundly; the next morning got up and felt fantastic. I felt so wonderful in that room that I actually made it my bedroom and spent the rest of my time in that home sleeping in a room that even non-allergic people found disgusting. People would go into that room and sneeze and cough and make suggestions about needing an ozone machine because it was so moldy.

When God delivers, it's supernatural; you just don't have that problem anymore. I had confronted deception and let it know that I would not be backed up. I would no longer be conned by the law. I would not hold back. My mentality had been changed. I was a victim no more ... I was a retaliator!

*Proverbs 3:5: "Trust in the Lord with all thine heart;*
*and lean not unto thine own understanding."*

Generational principalities will try to threaten a person who is gaining power by stepping out in faith. They will desire to instill fear with the warning voice of distraction, declaring, "You're going to lose everything."

When the "you're going to lose everything" voice is heard, it's time to take more. In other words, "don't hold back on me now" was the essence of what was happening: a primal interpretation, a spiritual reality. I was not moving ahead. I was being stalemated by a spiritual attack that I couldn't see.

I could see my kidneys, could feel my pain. I could hear fear and doubt. All of that was a mere distraction. That had nothing do with what was really going on spiritually. I was focused on one piece of land: the "new room." I had a faith agenda; I had to get a little bigger than my understanding.

The illusion of mold and dust allergy had been exposed. The attack of aggressive threats and their perceptions having power over me had been conquered.

# Chapter 29

## Take More Land

I knew that I had to continue to move forward, to press ahead. I was being made very cognizant of this "holding back syndrome" and how it could be detrimental to my health. My very life depended on it.

> Hebrews 10:38: "... but if any man draw
> back, my soul shall have no pleasure in him."

## Moving On

What was next? God had my full attention. I did not want to fall prey to mishap. I wanted to move ahead A.S.A.P. I had a land list. The next things that I had to deal with (take back) were the...

## Fourteen Teeth in My Mouth That Had No Fillings

During my illness, my last medical intervention before my total collapse was a dental escapade led by the law of sin and death, a misadventure of the curse itself! Generational principalities of wrathful idolatry had warred violently for my soul.

I had been diagnosed with mercury amalgam toxicity poisoning. There were many dentists and tests to validate this diagnosis. The laboratory tests resulted in thirty pages of mercury evaluation in the blood. These tests concluded quite clearly that removing all of the mercury from my mouth would be of tremendous benefit to me and probably lead to my entire healing.

My personal internist persuaded me to do this work. He was certain that mercury poisoning was my entire problem. He was convinced by the test results! He was elated to find the source of my misery and encouraged me to remove all mercury from my fillings. There was no doubt in my doctor's mind that this mercury toxicity was the cause of my environmental illness and immune suppression. He was certain that the cure would come from its removal.

This man had been my doctor since the inception of my illness. He tried many alternatives and conventional ways to get me well. He was an extremely caring man and had become a very good friend. I knew that he was sincere; this was not about making money. He truly believed that this would help me. He had spent a lot of his personal time researching what might help people like me with environmental illness.

I had been his first environmentally ill patient. Since then he had become very interested in the disease and turned his practice into a treatment center for the environmentally ill. He had gone to many environmental and immune dysfunction seminars where mercury toxicity removal was advocated; he felt strongly about it.

Many people claimed that they had gotten completely well after the mercury removal process. I cannot say that I shared his enthusiasm, but any hope, any attempt to solve my problem was welcomed at that time in my life! We went over all the tests; all the literature validated my doctor's research about the toxic mercury fillings.

## Lucky to Be Alive

We learned about all the illnesses that mercury could cause in the human body, destroying the entire immune system, lowering the t-cell count, and creating viruses in the blood. My personal test results were high; I was allergic and toxic from this mercury poisoning. According to the medical evaluations I was, in fact, lucky to be alive.

## The Amalgam Tattoo

There were other very evident manifestations of my poisoning. I had the mercury amalgam tattoo! The mercury tattoo is a sign, an omen—a diagnostic appendage to the mercury-testing arsenal. I had several of them — a clear-cut case of mercury poisoning. The mercury tattoo shows up near a filling. It is not on the actual tooth. It is a separate marking of the mercury metal itself. The gums surrounding the mercury-filled tooth turn blue. This tattoo-like discoloration is indicative of the poisoning. It is a red flag for a mercury poisoning diagnosis. It was evident to all: I had to have all the mercury removed as soon as possible.

## There Is a Dentist for Every Type of Dentistry

We had to hunt for this type of specialist. We didn't want a new kid on the mercury bandwagon; we wanted a seasoned believer.

## Electromagnetic Problems

This new dentist was very advanced; he had machines that could test for poisoning, that could even test for electrical malfunction in the mouth. My dental dilemmas were adding up. My new dentist found that I also had electromagnetic discrepancies in my mouth. My teeth were being polarized!

The new dental expert concluded that this negative polarization was affecting my brain, nervous and immune systems, throwing all my organs out of sync! He had huge charts, diagrams of every tooth and the corresponding organ that the tooth affected and had power to control.

For example, an upper right bicuspid would affect the lung organ; if this tooth had mercury in it or was electromagnetically compromised, it could destroy normal lung functioning. I was soon to realize my mercury toxicity dental problems were only the beginning of my woes. I also had severe electromagnetic disruptions, malfunctions, deriving from an old implant. I actually had one of the first dental implants ever put in a mouth. I had had it done experimentally (free), at the USC dental clinic when I was in college. It was a successful implant; I received it well and never had a problem with it. It held a space for two missing teeth and without it I had no left lower quadrant to chew with.

## Take It Out

It would be a small sacrifice, I was told, to get my health back. I could not eat anyhow! The removal of these implants for electrical restoration purposes was also in the experimental stage. I was lucky enough to have a dentist who was well versed in all of these new scientific environmental strategies.

The implant had a blade. The blade was about three-quarters deep into the gum area. It was lodged deep in my tissues; it had been in there a long time. I had heard that some of the original implants had been rejected, but mine was in there strong; it had become a part of my mouth. The implant involved three teeth: the one that it was next to and the two that it replaced, and it had crowns over it. All of this had to be surgically removed. I agreed to the operation.

I then had another situation to deal with. I could not have anesthesia. This was about detoxing, not adding toxicity. How were we to remove this life-threatening implant without anesthesia? There was no nontoxic way to do this; I would have to do it cold turkey.

## Mercury Removal

My dentist thought we should take out the mercury first. Fourteen teeth were stripped of all the amalgam fillings. I was sent home. I felt so weird; there were even a couple in the front that had fillings removed, fillings that were in the back, hidden, holding crowns together. The crowns also had to be removed. I now had two stubs for front teeth. It was not very attractive. Not that I was going anywhere, and of course, it would soon be replaced with less toxic materials. It was temporary and could save my life. I accepted this and went home feeling hopeful.

I couldn't look in the mirror; I was starting to not look like myself! I was beginning to take on the appearance of someone who could not afford dental work. Taking out the fillings and removing the crowns was more expensive than putting them in, but it gave me a desperate and destitute look. I looked very poor; I was dressed shabbily, in nontoxic attire, and now I had no teeth.

The dentist and my doctor encouraged me. *It will soon be over*, they agreed. *We will move ahead and take out all the crowns and the implant that is creating the electromagnetic dysfunction. You will be a new woman soon*, I was told. They were expecting this healing to come very soon, with all that electromagnetic pressure taken off and all the toxic mercury amalgam removed. I was on my way to health restoration.

I did not feel better after the mercury removal. Instead, I felt much worse. I was told that I wouldn't feel better till my mouth was restored electromagnetically. Then my progress would all kick in. I made my next appointment to have the implant removed.

## Shaking, Blue and Cold

I drove to the dental office that morning hopeful that I would get my life back. The operation was more than I had bargained for. My body went into trauma; the implant was lodged deeper than it had appeared on the x-ray. It became major surgery.

I started shaking from head to toe, and the dentist was afraid to give me anesthesia due to my allergies. I almost went unconscious with pain. I didn't actually pass out, I just shook. My body got ice cold and went into an involuntary shaking, like a bird about to expire. I shook and shook. I actually went into shock, turned blue, and then the operation was over.

## I Went Home to Die

When I went home that day, I went home to die. That was it. It was my last procedure, the last dentist, and the last doctor. My last chance at getting well.

I went so far down after that, I became so chemically intolerant, that I was unable to leave my "safe" house to even attempt to get help, and no one was able to enter. Every day I got worse, more sensitive, more allergic to everything. At first, it seemed like I was just in the process of recovering from the operation ...

## Then, When I Just Couldn't Get Back on My Feet

At first, I believed that during the mercury removal procedure, some of the toxic mercury had seeped into my bloodstream creating more toxicity. That was the dental rationale. Then, there was the "healing crisis" theory. "Of course, there are symptoms of getting worse before you get better," I was told. A healing crisis, I have discovered, is a term employed when no one wants to take responsibility for their actions! When you are getting worse, not better, no healing in sight, the spirit of self-justification generally sounds something like this: "Oh, you're really doing great. You're just going through a healing crisis!"

They meant that, even though I was getting sicker, even if I might be dying, was unable to sleep, eat, or leave my home—that was still a positive report. I was just in a temporary changing-of-the-guards state of flux. Healing was on the way. Healing was stalling, but would soon manifest! Eventually, what went from medical enthusiasm (everyone's certainty that I would experience a total healing) became a waiting game, and then a disappearing act.

The unconscious guilt from this type of inhumane experience is hard for any person to consciously acknowledge.

It soon became obvious that I was not in a healing crisis. I was in a "hanging on for dear life" crisis. I was in a "what in God's name happened here" crisis! I was in total confusion, total oppression, and total fatigue. I was in a "down as you could get and still be alive" crisis.

# Chapter 30

## What Really Happened

I will share with you (for anyone that has ever had a surgery or any unnecessary medical procedure), to clarify for every human heart and spirit, every reader, the danger of giving our power to the medical profession. I will tell you what really happened.

## My Barometer of Righteousness

If truth is light and light is revelation given by God, then when I walk towards God, I will have more aliveness. I have more light, my spirit is upheld. *"... the Lord upholds the righteous." (Isaiah 41:13)* It is a natural thing.

*Romans 8:10: "The Spirit is life because of righteousness."*

When my spirit is in control, as God created it, I have all the fruits of the spirit. It is who I am. I don't have to beg for it, tithe for it, pray for it, or fast for it. I am it!

I am the righteousness of God, the spirit person, with Divine health! Our spirits must control our hearts. The mind of the spirit must overcome the carnal mind with the truth. That is health. *"But if ye be led of the Spirit, ye are not under the law." (Galatians 5:18)*

## The Law of Sin and Death

To be under the law is to be in the curse. The curse of the law brings death; its roots are in idolatry. The law of sin and death (sin consciousness) is simply the consciousness or awareness of guilt and condemnation. It's the generationally inherited consciousness of victimization and disconnection from God.

We are in a very active battle with the law of sin and death versus the Perfect Law of Liberty. In every problem we face in our daily lives, this battle is at the core. Our freedom in Christ opposes the law of religion. We are always in a battle with the spirit of condemnation and guilt versus forgiveness and grace.

The battle is the Lord's when it is fought from the truth of the spirit. (1 Samuel 17:47, 2 Chronicles 20:15) When you are in the real battle, you will be raised up to perceive in spiritual integrity the condemnation and guilt that the law would use to steal your grace.

We must identify freedom and separate it from the law of sin and death. Then we will no longer be deceived by this evil quenching of God's Perfect Law of Liberty! His grace is sufficient!

*2 Corinthians 12:9: "And He said unto me, 'My grace is sufficient for thee: for my strength is made perfect in weakness.' "*

I believe that what the Lord meant when he said to Paul, "My grace is sufficient for thee"—was and is exactly that: "sufficient." It is enough. It covers your situation. It covers your personal thorn. You have it! You are healed!

Take it and enforce His grace. Enforcing His grace is true worship to God.

We are fighting to see above darkness, to discern truth from error, flesh from spirit, God's will from the carnal mind. (1 John 4:6)

If we are privileged in Christ to see this basic primal battle for what it is, we can deal with it directly, take our rightful authority. All of our other (alleged) problems will be dissipated. *They are just symptoms of this battle between the flesh and the spirit.*

*Romans 8:13: "For if ye live after the flesh, ye shall die ..."*

## The Real Problem

I had a problem; my problem was I had been deceived by beliefs of dentists, medical diagnoses, and other assorted opinions of the world. This does not mean that all dentists and doctors are insincere. This simply means that many times they themselves are deceived. They are looking at the problem thinking that you are your body, as if your body controls you!

When we understand that we are spiritual beings, potentially controlled by grace, we see things differently. We begin to take on a spiritual perspective. We as believers can grow and deepen in our wisdom in this area.

## A Spiritual Diagnosis

I was in a spiritual battle! My old nature was on a roll and had taken control of my spirit. My spirit had been assaulted, brought under subjection by the impostor; now my spirit was fighting for its authority!

My destiny, my purpose, was not being realized. I was dying of spiritual oppression, of powerlessness. I did not have enough light in my body to survive. I wasn't getting any light from treatments. Every time I had another medical or dental "treatment," my heart, my spirit, grew more confused, progressively withdrawn, hopeless, losing light, truth, power and righteousness. Soon, I was on empty. I had fallen off the track of destiny. I had fallen prey to vultures.

*John 6:63: "It is the spirit that quickeneth; the flesh profiteth nothing."*

## A Carnal Con Job

All of my symptoms had absolutely nothing to do with my teeth, my body, electromagnetic energy, mercury toxicity, the air, etc. These were all distractions, self-justifications of the carnal nature, and fake symptoms of the impostor (carnal mind) itself. The impostor had set me up to take me out (of my destiny). It was sabotaging my inevitable power over it by distracting me into a medical perspective, deceiving me to believe that I was, in fact, my body. It was doing what it does best, trying to save itself by luring me into further procrastination of my dominion.

## I Am Not My Body

I am not matter; I am spirit. How could matter heal me? I could only be deceived by matter impersonating me, lulling me into denial and leading me astray. Once I was misled, I could be more easily seduced into bowing to its generational idols. Then, evil could give me its second punch — to blame me, condemn me, and punish me for its error. This is the lack of forgiveness of the law. The less light I had, the more condemnation I would be receptive to. The more condemnation and guilt, the more oppression I had.

The more oppression I had (spirit overcome by law), the more power it had to deceive me. In buying this material diagnosis, I had identified myself with the perceptions of the flesh, and with it, the ways of the law. I was, in fact, agreeing with the oppressor of my spirit. I had lost my separation from evil, my reality, and had embraced the impostor's illusions. Here was its evil goal fulfilled, the relinquishment of my proper identity. My position of righteousness had been the target all along!

*Romans 7:24: "Who will rescue me from the body of this death?"*

*Psalm 18:20: "The Lord rewarded me according to my righteousness."*

# Lawful Opportunist

The opposition could not touch me on Holy Ground! Holy Ground was led by God. The generational mind first had to knock me off balance, and then mislead me, in order to attack. Once I was led astray, tossed off my path, it could begin to inflict one deception after another. There would be a literal downward spiral of guilt personified. To receive the guilt, I would have to relinquish my grace (forgiveness). I would have to make a conscious choice: guilt or grace. With a guilt choice, the law would prevail and its curse flourish, blossoming and rejoicing while it had an opportunity to kick me while I was down.

The law of sin and death warred aggressively against me. I had forgotten who I was. Evil, however, had eternal recall and wanted to keep me in darkness.

# Chapter 31

## The Natural Perspective (Material Consciousness) (How It Manifested in My World and Body)

I became more sensitive and much more allergic to food and to the environment. I could no longer get out of bed. I could no longer walk outside my home. I had become so weakened by deception, so acutely environmentally ill, that every germ, virus, fume, mold spore, every chemical, and every energy on earth had power over me.

## Biblical Perspective (Tossed)

*Ephesians 4:14: "That we henceforth be no more children, tossed to and fro, and carried about with every wind of doctrine, by the sleight of men, and cunning craftiness, whereby they lie in wait to deceive."*

## That's What Happened to Me: I Was Tossed

My original problem was being tossed and deceived by error moving through people, creating idols via codependency. In my pursuit of health, I was just tossed more! I was discovering the medical toss to be a grander scheme of evil than the relationship toss.

I was not solving my problem of "being tossed," but adding to it! That's why I became sicker with each treatment. The problem was not the solution. Of course, in retrospect that is all very clear, but in the midst of it, Lord have mercy!

I had not taken care of myself. The revelation that the Lord would eventually give me, the revelation that would raise me from the dead, needed to be implemented. My emotional and spiritual integrity had been compromised! It was a deep blow to my heart.

> *Romans 8:28: "And we know that all things work together for good to them that love God, to them who are the called according to his purpose."*

> *Psalm 103:4: "Who redeemeth thy life from destruction; who crowneth thee with lovingkindness and tender mercies."*

## The Real Solution (Retaliate)
## (The Land of Mercury Toxicity and
## Other Dental and Medical Illusions)

There I was: new house, new foods, and fourteen teeth with no fillings from the mercury removal rampage! I was left with fourteen teeth with huge holes. I had to let go of my former dental beliefs and replace these fillings by faith. Teeth were next on my list. I couldn't avoid it any longer! I did not want to indulge the "holding back syndrome."

I chose the one dentist who would not involve himself in the "mercury toxicity escapade." He had refused to partake in the mercury removal plan; he didn't feel that I had the strength to go through the procedure at that time. He didn't believe it to be a proper solution for my dilemma. As you can only imagine, dentists were not popular with me at this time in my life. I had to trust one to fill my teeth.

### Now I Know It's God

Dr. Carter examined my teeth, then turned to me and remarked, "Juliana, I don't know how to tell you this, but there have been so many years with no fillings in your mouth, all

**203**

your teeth have shifted and there are huge spaces in between them. Ordinarily, I would use gold, porcelain or ceramic composites; however, in your situation, the only alloy that could hold your teeth together is mercury.

"I am sorry to have to tell you this," Dr. Carter went on. "The irony of the situation is that the only way I can effectively fill these teeth is by putting in three times the amount of mercury in your teeth that you originally had."

"Unfortunately," Dr. Carter cringed as he made this next statement, "this will be all brand-new mercury. I don't even like to work with it myself. There is no other option! It is the only way to fill holes of that size!"

## Bravo, Jesus

I found myself amused. Three times the amount of original mercury! I laughed. It was a cosmic joke, a heavenly ha-ha! *I have come full circle*, I thought. *God must be showing me how ridiculous this whole concept is and I'm going to prove it by putting in three times the original amount of mercury in my mouth.* I was laughing in the joy of the Lord! God Himself was upping the ante, destroying illusions. This was to be a grand Divine Retaliation! Three times the amount of brand-new, reeking mercury! Bravo, Jesus!

I responded to my dentist, "Dr. Carter, that's great news. I am certain that God is in agreement!" I left, making the appointment to have a quarter of my mouth filled with brand new mercury amalgam.

## D (Dentist) Day

The day came for me to go to the dental office. I drove around the block three times with such high anxiety that I couldn't even find the building. Finally I found it, somehow managed to park my car, and went inside.

## Between God and Me

I didn't share all the problems I'd had after the mercury removal with my dentist because I knew that he would not want to be involved in the mercury replacement if he knew my history. This was between God and me. There was no Nellie in the wings. I was growing up. I knew that the Son of God had the authority to forgive sin! (Matthew 9:6)

## This Time, God Was in Control

I sat listening to my praise music — speakers over my ears, smelling mercury fumes, hearing drills, and soon it was over. You could sense the presence of God in the room; there was a supernatural flow. I had no pain; I didn't need novocaine then and never have in any dental work since. This time, God was in control. I was led. There was nothing I could do but wait. I went home and felt pretty good. I simply and calmly went to bed and got up the next morning. Chop wood. Carry water. Christian style.

> *Psalm 78:35: "And they remembered that God was their rock, and the high God their redeemer."*

# Chapter 32

## The Next Morning

I had always had a lingering back pain from my illness. I often wore a back brace. That morning, when I arose, I forgot to put on the back brace because my back felt fine. I didn't understand the connection between back pain and adding mercury to my teeth. Why would my back be improved from adding mercury? There was, of course, no connection between my teeth and my back, except my barometer of righteousness. My faith, my power and integrity had been increased and my body was following.

Deceptions had been eliminated, and error had been overcome. I had more healing. I learned one thing over and over; you can't get healed from what doesn't exist. Proper identification is power in the spiritual realm. If there is no such thing as mercury toxicity, you can't get healed from removing it. I did, however, get healed from God's plan of Divine Retaliation: the counterattack of upping the ante and the demonstration of faith — the action of putting all the mercury back in. Three times the amount of mercury had a lot of retaliation faith power.

> 2 Samuel 22:21: "The Lord rewarded me
> according to my righteousness: according to the
> cleanness of my hands hath he recompensed me."

## Mercury Beliefs Attempted to Toss Me

There were temptations during the week after the mercury replacement. As I went about my business and touched things around my house, I experienced an additional sensitivity, as if I were having toxic reactions to everything. My carnal mind would continuously remind me how toxic mercury was, and that I had added layers of deadly toxicity.

"It's new mercury," it would remind me, "brand new, much more toxic than the old mercury that has already outgassed," it aggressively suggested daily. "You should have it all taken out."

Yeah, right!

## Upping the Ante

There was really nothing to war about.

> *2 Corinthians 10:3: "For though we walk*
> *in the flesh, we do not war after the flesh."*

Been there, done that. I knew that warring wouldn't resolve anything. I decided to move ahead by faith. I made a decision to put all the mercury back in my mouth.

More mercury would solve these minor irritations. This effort of oppressing me into "fear of" reactions would soon be retaliated. I identified the spirit of self-justification, which was pointing a finger at toxins, distracting me from my truth. The enemies of our true essence will always direct us into medical or psychological thinking, throwing a curve ball to take us into denial. Denial is less light; denial is darkness.

## It's the Thought that Counts

The deceptive thought is always pointing a finger at something other than the lie in your mind that is really creating the symptom in your body. I was learning how to handle darkness.

> *Acts 26:18: "To open their eyes, and to turn them from*
> *darkness to light, and from the power of Satan unto God,*
> *that they may receive forgiveness of sins, and inheritance*
> *among them which are sanctified by faith that is in me."*

## More Mercury Coming Up

I continued in my Divine Retaliation. I made another appointment and filled another quadrant of teeth with mercury. I was doing the threatening. If I received any reaction after my dental appointments, I made another appointment as soon as possible.

My symptoms were always resolved by an additional dose of brand new mercury. Three times the amount! Things were rapidly changing. Now, instead of fear-related reactions, I would be euphoric. If I wanted to feel great, all I had to do was go have some dental work. It was as if God had taken over. My dentist was now reconstructing crowns and completing the total restoration of my teeth. I felt no pain. I had no novocaine. The dentist was amazed.

I was in a palpable, miraculous move of God.

## Another Idol Bites the Dust (The Mercury)

*It is ridiculous enough,* I thought, *that I bought this mercury toxicity concept on a level of common sense.* To see it exposed as a total scam of evil was edifying to my soul. A large healing came from this mercury retaliation — more energy, more aliveness, more faith, more righteousness, and additional proper identity. Another idol had been overcome.

*1 John 5:21: "Little children, keep yourselves from idols. Amen."*

## Less Tossed

I now had normal teeth. I was able to chew properly. I had food, and I could eat, chew, and digest. I could smile and be presentable. I had a normal house that I was able to live in. I was wearing normal clothes. This was huge for someone who had been dying and hopeless just a few short months ago! A dream come true! This didn't happen because of years of medical treatments. It was the exact opposite of that. I was undoing medical treatments. I was in the process of laying every idol down. This was not a slow or gradual recovery. I had only been on my Retaliation journey for three and one-half months and I was feeling great!

This was just the beginning of a life of faith.

I relaxed, took a deep breath and started to enjoy living in a real house. I began to go out in the community and connect with others.

My house was a six-month rental. The owners would be returning soon, and it would be time for me to move on. It had been a wonderful time for me. I had gained a lot of territory and had much victory. I lived in peace for the first time in years!

# Chapter 33

## The Next Move

I was between moves. I knew that God wanted me to move back to Los Angeles — the perfect place to live for an environmentally concerned person who was stepping out in faith. Los Angeles had it all: smog, pollen, traffic, and mass humanity. It was a toxic paradise. It also had more life, and life was what I was taking back.

## There Is an Appointed Time for Every Purpose (Ecclesiastes 3:1)

I wasn't sure if my time in Santa Barbara was up yet. I stayed one more season in laid-back Santa Barbara, and God honored it.

## The Last Santa Barbara House

A door had opened. A door had shut. My decision was made, and I moved into the next Santa Barbara house. I was to continue to retaliate.

## The Next Stand

There were rooms in this home that I could go into, and there were rooms that I couldn't even walk near! I had more chemical tolerance from my last victory, and much more stamina and spiritual power.

There was one room in the home with new carpet — a brand new carpet that had just been installed the day before. The landlords believed that they were doing me a favor! It reeked of formaldehyde, that new carpet smell! I shut the door to the new carpet disaster and proceeded to use the rest of the house.

## Taking the Formaldehyde New Carpet Room (The Laying Down of Another Idol)

Formaldehyde is considered to be a huge environmental hazard for a compromised immune system and to all allergy sufferers. It is claimed by many to be a very dangerous chemical. It outgasses deadly fumes. Many people had gotten environmental illness from formaldehyde exposures alone.

## Attacked in the Room

Every time I walked into the room with the new carpet, my whole body went into spasms, and I got a headache. There was nothing I knew that I could do to stop these reactions. I had to avoid the room or ruin my day.

## A Spiritual Sense

I decided to make that room a place of worship. I would give it to God. I would turn the possessed room into a sanctuary unto the Lord Himself! If I couldn't live in it, I would not let it go to waste. I was tired of giving up territory, tired of wasted space, of closing doors, living in fear of this and fear of that.

*1 Peter 5:17: "Casting all your care upon Him; for he careth for you."*

## Preparing a Sanctuary

Each day I would go in and add things. I was decorating a sanctuary, preparing an offering unto the Lord. I made beautiful white doilies and covered and decorated furniture. I created a handmade altar with beautiful red satin and velvet pillows. Every day, I handpicked flowers from my daily nature walks, each one chosen by the Lord Himself.

Everything in the room was a sacrifice, a thought, a feeling, a consecration—a worship unto God. It reflected an appreciation for all that I had: Everything that I had was given to me by God. I wanted to show my gratefulness, to give back. My heart was full of love for my Savior, and I wanted to marry Him, be His bride, which I, of course, was. But I wanted a ceremony, something romantic, intimate. Every day I added something — more candles, more gifts. I added it slowly, lovingly, with great care, with passion, as one would caress a lover. I was making love to Christ.

*1 Chronicles 16:29: "Worship the Lord in the beauty of holiness."*

*Psalm 95:6: "O come, let us worship and bow down: let us kneel before the Lord our maker."*

## The Room Gets New Life

The vibration in the room started to build; the room began to have a life of its own. The energy of the room started to change. The room itself had become anointed as if there was someone living in it. It became tangibly apparent that there was supernatural activity going on in there. The atmosphere of the room was strangely intense, and the anointing was escalating daily!

I could now go in and worship pleasantly for about fifteen minutes. I would then leave, but not run or walk fast to get out. Each day I needed less recovery time. I was being upheld in the anointing of the room itself. The room had become illuminated.

It had beautiful glass candle lamps hanging from the walls. The room seemed lit up, even when there were not any candles or lights turned on. "The room" had become a very special place. We were having a grand time together, the King of the Universe and I. I went shopping for my wedding gown.

## Katrina Gets Slain

I spent a few hours each day going in and out of the room, decorating it and avoiding reactions. It was an ongoing project.

Katrina, a spiritual sister from Los Angeles, came for a visit. She didn't know I had made the "new carpet room" a place of worship. I had not shared that fact or shown the room to anyone. She asked me to show her this room I had been decorating. She walked into "the room."

## Katrina Is Slain in the Spirit

Katrina was actually slain in the spirit! The anointing in that room had become extremely powerful. It had the kind of anointing a congregation gets after a week of dedicated and consecrated praise, fasting and worship — a revival anointing. Katrina had spiritual gifts and sensitivity and was a consecrated student in the spirit of God. We shared God together and had that extra bonding of the spiritually sensitive.

She walked into the room and fell down; she was slain in the spirit. "This has never happened to me before, Juliana," Katrina exclaimed. "I have never felt an anointing that strong in my life. Did someone get healed in there? What is going on in there?" she wanted to know.

Katrina confirmed my suspicions that there was something going on spiritually and supernaturally in that room. I didn't tell her that I was romancing the Lord; it seemed too personal at the time, a sacred intimacy. I think she suspected!

## I Still Had Reactions

Every day in "the room," I lit candles, changed water for the plants and flowers, added little things, worshipped, praised the Lord and got out. I could still feel the formaldehyde affecting my body. I was still reacting to the room. I was preparing the room for something. I was not there yet. I did not have the victory from decorating the room, nor did I have a revelation on what to do next.

## The Wedding Night

Finally, I felt it was time. The sanctuary was complete. I decided that I would just go and sleep in the room, which had apparently been positioned to have its own life. I felt led, beckoned to take it on, in a different way. An unusual type of stand!

I put on my beautiful, white nightgown wedding dress and filled the room with handpicked bridal flowers. I put on my gold wedding band that the Lord had chosen for me on one of our outings. I went into the room and gave the whole situation to God. I just stayed in the room. I slept in the room that I could not safely walk in and out of! I married the Lord that night. I was blissfully happy.

## The Bride of Christ (Revelation 21:2)

I woke up the next morning married to Jesus. There was never another reaction to that room again or to any other new carpet anywhere. I was totally delivered. I realized once again that things are not what they appear to be.

I was learning more about God's ways of healing. My education in healing was very tangible, because my illness included an immediate reaction to chemicals and foods. Environmental illness had a way of magnifying physical illusions more than another type of disease. All illnesses are, of course, based in similar illusions — inherited and contrived deceptions of the generational mind.

I was learning that illness itself could not survive in a system of faith. If faith was higher than error or disharmony, a person could be healed. Faith would lead a person to the truth. Of course, if you had the truth to begin with, you would not need to be healed. You would be the recipient of Divine health. Positive thinking does not have spiritual power; it is mental ascent. It is mostly the carnal mind conning you into a pie-in-the-sky hype, but cleverly keeping you in its realm, its jurisdiction, in the law. There is no grace in it. Grace is a spiritual attribute. Faith itself will guide someone to take their proper position as *"... the head and not the tail of their own body." (Deuteronomy 28:13)*

# Chapter 34

## Idols of "Fear Of"

Illness is based on deception. Deception needs a person to bow to it in order to oppress their spirit. Usually deception uses "fear of" something. "Fear of" is an idol of the carnal mind, its kingpin.

> Mark 3:27: "No man can enter into a strong man's house, and spoil his goods, except he will first bind the strong man; and then he will spoil his house."

It is a system of mind control. Entertaining "fear of" anything will put your mind in a jam and toss you into your own personalized unconscious generational principality hell. "Fear of" has many different twists and deceptions!

## The Past

"Fear of" can be used to re-stimulate old behaviors, old triggers, and old ways. The triggers do not belong to you; they are invented from the "old creatures," generational past. These triggers are perceived askew, not unlike the political propaganda of slanted crisis news reporting. They are the perceptions of guilt and unholiness. To focus on them is to perpetuate disempowerment. The perceptions of the carnal mind are used to justify its existence and distract you from your reality.

## New Creature/New Town

In Christ, we are healed because we are no longer subject to the old creature. We are translated into being spirit. The spirit person has the capacity to separate from the old creature and the "fear of" manipulations of the mind control system.

These old patterns, if not identified and brought under subjection by the spirit, will rule us. Unidentified deceptions via thoughts can shut our hearts, leaving us feeling numb and passionless. That is the plan of evil: our hearts hardened and numb!

God's plan is for us to connect deeply with each other from our heart of hearts—deeply and authentically. Love covers a multitude of sins, and love fulfills the law. We have been born into an inheritance that has given us dominion over all of these alleged human ailments. They are not at all what we call them or what we have been taught to perceive them to be.

To stay ahead of this generationally inherited past, one has to live as the spirit person.

God was leading me back to Los Angeles, the City of Angels, to do just that!

> *2 Corinthians 5:17: "Therefore if any man be*
> *in Christ, he is a new creature: old things are*
> *passed away; behold, all things are become new."*

Los Angeles would be a profoundly wonderful land to conquer next. It was time to go home to a real city, to a place with serious challenges. Huge challenges for me! L.A. was a retaliator's graduate school of the spirit — a place conducive to advanced battles.

## A Toxic Hell

Los Angeles is renowned for being one of the most toxic cities in the world — the car fumes, chemical spills, the smog, and constant pesticide spraying everywhere. L.A. is definitely an environmentally unconscious town. No one with environmental illness has ever chosen or been advised to move there. The environmentally ill community in L.A. was warned to get out as soon as possible, to run for the hills! In the immune-compromised world, it was "run to the desert and clean, dry air."

*1 Corinthians 1:27: "But God hath chosen the*
*foolish things of the world to confound the wise."*

## Moving Back to Los Angeles

This next move was done in a rush. I had looked all over the city, searched and searched. And, I must confess, I was intimidated. I found it hard to make a decision. The crowds, the barking dogs—there was always something. Finally, I had stalled so long that I was starting to have physical symptoms. I wasn't moving, and my bowels weren't, either. I knew I was in trouble. I have noticed that the bowels of man and the heart are synonymous in the spirit. To me, bowel dysfunction was generally an indication that I was moving in a wrong direction, out of purpose. In this case, I was literally not moving at all!

My current situation inspired me to let go of the hunt for the perfect place and move as quickly as I could. I grabbed an immediately available furnished apartment.

*Lamentations 1:20: "Behold, O Lord; for I am in distress:*
*my bowels are troubled; mine heart is turned within me ..."*

## Wilshire Blvd., Westwood
## (One of the Busiest Streets in the World)

The apartment that I moved into A.S.A.P. was in a huge condominium building on Wilshire Blvd. This would be my first big city living in a long time. I had not lived in such close proximity to other human beings in eighteen years. I chose this place only because it was immediately available. The traffic on Wilshire was unending; it was considered to be one of the most congested streets in the world!

At first, it was kind of exciting. Then I started to notice that my old town had changed. There were no American people in my building — a whole building with not one other American! The apartments were very close together. I could feel the energy from the other tenants come through the walls, hear their conversations, smell their foods cooking. Quite a change from wilderness living.

I was used to hearing birds chirp in my window in the mountains. Now I was hearing traffic noise and sirens. I was used to having gentle and beautiful deer look at me through my kitchen window every morning. I was now experiencing mothers of Jewish–Persian men accosting me in the elevator to inquire if I were first Jewish and then single. Times had changed.

## No Peace in Westwood

My nights were spent wide awake. I felt as if I lived in an emergency room in a hospital. The ambulance sirens screeched all night long. The close proximity to UCLA and other hospitals in the area kept the sirens roaring — always a soul in trauma, going to the hospital, getting emergency treatment.

The traffic roared twenty-four hours a day, seven days a week, without a break. The freeway whirled close by. Wilshire Blvd. was a major intersection and connected people to the beach, downtown, Century City, and Beverly Hills. I was living in the middle of mass humanity! The buses stopped on every corner throughout the night and began again early in the morning. There were no breaks, no peace.

My bedroom, I found out as I attempted to sleep, was right on top of the boiler room. The boiler room held all of the machines that powered the building. The boiler room noise was not a consistent hum, not a sound that one could grow accustomed to. There were twelve separate boilers that made their individual sounds. Not one hiss, but different hisses: loud hisses and clanging on and off; one would go on, another off, with different tones at different times.

I heard a variety of volumes, all inconsistent. I could not adjust to the sound; I could not play my music above it. It was like a large, out-of-tune band that could not play in harmony. It was louder, stranger, weirder than any other sound I'd heard; it had its own rhythm, its own beat. The only thing that could subdue the traffic noise was the boiler room clanging directly under my bedroom window!

I hadn't slept in an entire week, not for one moment! From the boiler room, there was hissing and spitting all night, along with traffic — tooting horns, screeching tires, fumes, and assorted bus sounds. I was exhausted, getting worn down. I could hardly think.

## Bad Council Inspiration

A minister friend of mine was having a meeting in Westwood. His church was not far from my new home. I went to the meeting and sought his council. "I know all about that problem," Pastor Bob said. "My wife Carol has trouble sleeping in the city; she wears earplugs. She puts them on before she goes to sleep and fills the room with praise music."

I had already tried the praise music plan; it was ineffective for me. My situation was different. I didn't want to hide. I wanted a faith solution. I felt undermined by the suggestion. Spiritual undermining was not God's plan. However, after thinking about his words for a while, I became inspired.

God wanted me to have another victory! I was here in L.A. to grow, to gain faith, not to put plugs in my ears. Although, to be honest, if it gave me a good night's sleep, I would have been glad to accept it. But it didn't, and it wouldn't! Often, bad advice was good for me. It would get me to feel and think differently. I had not come to L.A. to give up territory; I was here in Christ to take my land. As soon as I had that thought, I knew that I knew. I knew … what I had to do.

I started to think clearly, remembering that I was not to be pushed back like a victim. I had had enough of that. I began to think like a warrior. I started to think in faith. I would not bow to noise. God was God, and noise was noise, and I would have my peace wherever I was!

## I Would Retaliate

I would confront the situation; I would give it to God. I would not be backed down. I had not come this far to back down now. I was on a roll of faith! I would demonstrate His power! I would have my peace.

## Yes! Lord, Yes! (Mark 7:28)

I knew exactly what I had to do. I couldn't tell anyone; it would sound crazy. Tonight, I would not pull covers over my head, use headphones, music, earplugs, white noise, and shut windows and drapes tightly. No! This night I would not be led by apprehension and avoidance. This night, would be different! *I would take my peace, enforce my grace. I would demonstrate the victory of my King.*

## Come on In!

I went home that evening with a plan. The minute I opened my apartment door, I ran straight to the windows. They were tightly shut. I threw them open with a vengeance, opened them fully. I then threw the drapes open! I opened every sliding glass door in the living room! These glass doors were above the buses, traffic and fumes. I opened the doors as wide as I possibly could.

I was almost living in the street. I was only on the second floor! "Come on in!" I began screaming. "Come on in. You want to take my peace with your noise? You think my peace is dependent on noise? You ungodly fools! Bring your cars, trucks, buses, fumes, sirens. Bring more, bring it all on," I challenged as I continued to invite more noise in. I opened every window, every door. Anything that would enable noise to enter, I encouraged and opened.

I walked into my bedroom. As I did so, I felt my spirit rise up. My helper, the Holy Spirit, was with me. I had gotten God's attention; my faith would be honored and acknowledged!

I ran over to my windows above the boiler room and threw them open in a flash — bigger, wider, as large an opening as I could get. I opened the drapes, then opened the smaller windows on the other side of the room for a little extra traffic noise. This let in some extra siren drama. "Come on in! Come on in!" I was screaming like a mad woman. "Come on in. Make noise. Make your noise, all the noise you want, and then make more noise!" I was upping the ante on noise!

## More Noise!

This was not a time to get religious. This was a time to get down and dirty. I hadn't slept in a week! I opened everything I could find. I even turned on the fan in my little bathroom (it didn't have a window) just for some extra noise. Any little piece of noise I could get my hands on, I invited in. I was going somewhere; I was feeling it in the spirit. I had become righteously indignant, which was exactly where I needed to be! How dare any opposition to God come against the peace of His vessel!

I was retaliating from a position of righteousness, my position in Christ! I was, after all, the righteousness of God in Christ. Was I not given dominion on this earth over all things? I was. I knew I was. I knew that He did it. I knew that He gave it to me; I could not be convinced of anything else! Was I not promised a sweet sleep?

*Proverbs 3:24: "When thou liest down, thou shalt not be afraid: yea, thou shalt lie down, and thy sleep shall be sweet."*

## I Would Sleep on the Promise

It was a bizarre scenario — all the lights on, all the windows open. It looked as if someone was having a party on the terrace, which expanded into my fully opened and illuminated apartment. There did not appear to be a room in my apartment that would be conducive to sleep! I would sleep in utter chaos; I would sleep on the promise of sleep, not the atmosphere of my bedroom! I was moving spontaneously, beginning to feel satisfied, as if I had made my point, set my limits in the spirit world ...

I lay down on my bed and simply declared my position. "I am going to sleep." I was confident. I would give this to my Lord.

I then put my eyes on Jesus, connecting to the lover of my soul. "Lord, tomorrow I will have total peace, if I sleep or if I don't sleep! I will stay up tonight and praise you. I will praise you all night and feel great tomorrow. I will be refreshed; I cast this care on you." And then I did just that. I relaxed and decided to praise God all night. My heart was full of praise, and within minutes, I had fallen into a peaceful slumber.

*Isaiah 60:18: "Violence shall no more be heard in thy land, wasting nor destruction within thy borders; but thou shalt call thy walls Salvation and thy gates Praise."*

## Did I Imagine This?

I slept like a baby all night. When I awakened, it was ten in the morning. I had slept twelve hours. I could not hear the boiler room noise! The traffic noise was minimized! I could hear it, but

223

it didn't bother me; it was much lower, tolerable … It had lost its power to disrupt my peace!

The boiler room noise had ceased. The twelve boilers were totally silent. How could they be stopped? Did I imagine them? Had I finally cracked? I called two friends who had witnessed the boiler room noise; they couldn't stand it either. One friend of mine had tried to sleep over to comfort me. She had been driven out in the middle of the night by the boiler room noise. I invited her back.

## What Happened?

Gloria returned to my apartment, walked into the bedroom, opened the windows and said, "Where did it go? How can it be gone? I don't hear the boilers hissing! That was the loudest noise I had ever heard! No one could sleep with that irritating sound! What stopped it? What did you do? Tell me the truth, did you get the building to shut that awful noise down?"

# Chapter 35

## I Had My Promised Sweet Sleep

From that night on, in that bedroom I slept better than I had ever slept in my life. Nothing bothered me. I was unaware of any noise. I was totally protected from the disturbance. I had done my part, upped the ante, and called the bluff of deception. I showed my hand. I had the trump card. I had the power of God on my side. I could raise the stakes when I wanted and needed to raise them. I had rights, and I had backup on high to protect them. His grace was enforced!

*Exodus 15:6: "Thy right hand, O Lord, is become glorious in power: thy right hand, O Lord, hath dashed in pieces the enemy."*

I stayed peacefully on Wilshire Blvd. for a while and then moved to a comfortable home in a quieter area. God began to call me to minister to others.

## I Thought This Was about Faith

This was a time when the Lord was teaching me my ministry, preparing me for His service. I was thrilled to be asked to minister at a private home meeting. It would be my first solo ministry.

I was excited to serve the Lord and planned what I would say. I was very serious about being exact; I wanted to communicate God's truth without error. I had about ten pages of index cards — reminders, notes, prompters, and revelations. This was to be my first gig as a minister!

I was fully prepared. I was leaving my home to go to the meeting, and as I opened my car door to take off, the Lord spoke to me ... a word that I really didn't want to hear.

"I thought this was about faith," the Lord questioned.

I knew exactly what God meant. I got it intuitively, immediately; my old nature was stalling, buying time, making believe that this comment wasn't spoken. Perhaps if this comment were ignored, my old nature could follow the impostor's original agenda. I had spent a lot of time formulating my ministry plan of attack.

## Okay, Lord

"Of course it's about faith, Lord," I replied. "That's why I am going in faith. I am going to my first gig, my new ministry, in faith."

There was no response, no negotiating, no deal making.

I threw the index cards out of my car window, laughed, and agreed with God, seeing the intent of the law. "Okay, Lord, it's about faith. I will go with nothing, and your Holy Spirit will lead me and speak through me.

> Isaiah 49:2: "And He hath made my mouth like a
> sharp sword; in the shadow of His hand hath
> he hid me, and made me a polished shaft ..."

## The Ministry Led by God Is in the Moment

Ministers in Christ are in the moment of God, in the Kingdom of God, led by the Spirit of God to do His will.

I was a new minister. I wanted to be prepared for anything that might happen! God wanted to show me where my real power was. Not in elegant, prepared speeches, not in my knowledge, not even in God-given revelations — my power was in doing nothing but being led. There is an appointed time for every purpose unto heaven, and only God knew what would occur. It was a know-as-you-go opportunity and an on-the-job training program combined, all wrapped up in God's call.

Jeremiah 15:16: *"For I am called by thy name,*
*O Lord God of hosts."*

Romans 8:28: *"And we know that all things work*
*together for good to them that love God, to them*
*who are the called according to His purpose."*

## On-the-Job Training

That first night on the job, I was led to pray for people. I will never forget it. I put my hand on a woman's face that had an enlarged red wound with a tumor that stuck straight out like a cylinder-shaped boil.

The tumor came off in my hand!

I had not done anything but begin to pray — no casting, confessing or preaching. I put my hand on her face, and a tumor fell off in my hand. I didn't know what to do with it. I actually screamed and dropped it! Everyone laughed in the joy of the Lord.

The woman was healed!

It had been a cancerous tumor, and the woman's doctor wanted to remove it. She had refused the surgery, believing in God for her miracle! We all rejoiced and spent the rest of the evening praying, worshipping and praising the Lord.

## My Unprepared Gig

There were many healings that very first night; none of them had anything to do with me or the preparation of the carnal mind. The agenda of the flesh would have quenched the entire evening and all of God's miracles.

> *1 Corinthians 2:4: "And my speech and my preaching was not with enticing words of man's wisdom, but in demonstration of spirit and power."*

I learned that grace for ministry was by faith and faith only. Faith that God will show up and do something. It was about tarrying, just waiting on the Lord.

## The Agenda Quench

The Lord wanted me to realize that speaking from the agenda of notes was the carnal mind's plan — the impostor wanting to look important and intelligent—to imitate what it thought looked good. It wanted to impress people! When the spirit of God is not leading the ministry, the power of God is being stolen from God's vessels. While we are brilliantly prepared and being entertaining, reading our agenda, God is directing us, speaking to us, and giving us His plan.

I have never been embarrassed waiting on God; I have ministered when I have been low, sleepless, sans anointing, sans preparation, prayer and Bible reading. It has seemed to me that the worse shape I was in, the best I have gotten of God.

Folks, just relax and don't let your opposition condemn you into having to be somewhere special in your heart, your spirit, emotions, or even your faith. Enjoy the fact you can just do what God is asking you to do.

> *2 Corinthians 12:19: "… My strength is made perfect in weakness."*

## The Law and the Church

Many of God's men and women today in ministry are in a belief system of disempowerment and victimization—sin consciousness. This is what God wants to correct. When we take our rightful God-given place of spiritual authority, the church will become the hospital!

Those who know who they are in Him have His authority, and total dominion on this earth. These vessels combined, standing together in His authority, will have the power to heal hearts, minds and bodies all over the world! These consecrated servants will have His full capacity to see truth and not be deceived.

*John 14:12: "And greater works than these shall he do ..."*

It is the will of God at this time to empower His body. We will be brought together (knit together in love), (Colossians 2:2) and we will reign over deception on earth. We will stand with each other in truth, faith and purpose. We have already been healed."

*Isaiah 53:5: "And with his stripes we are healed."*

*1 Peter 2:24: "By whose stripes ye were healed."*

## The Healing Inheritance
## (Matthew 10:8, 1 Corinthians 12:28)

The Son of God has been given power to forgive sins! This forgiveness was and is the healing of your body, mind and heart! If you are not experiencing it, throw the deception out of your mind, bust the con, and enforce your God-given grace. Choose to live in total power on this earth! Your inheritance in Christ is complete!

There is absolutely nothing you have to do but walk fully in it.

# Chapter 36

## Additional Tales of Divine Retaliation

I am going to share a few stories for clarification of the simplicity of "Divine Retaliation."

I think it is best taught by testimony.

*1 Peter 1:19: "But with the precious blood of Christ, as of a lamb without blemish and without spot."*

*Revelation 12:11: "And they overcame him by the blood of the lamb, and by the word of their testimony ..."*

## The Smelly Green Cherokee

When I left Santa Barbara, I was driving an old beat-up (nontoxic, of course) Nissan, desirable because of its very beat-up condition. Like every possession that belongs to an environmentally ill person, it was a hand-me-down, hanging by a thread — an old, used, and rejected vehicle. I drove it by faith. It had 240,000 miles on it, but at least it had no "new car smell"! It was a car that I believed I could chemically tolerate. A decrepit car that would be suitable for my allergies would take me months to find, requiring much research and many horrible reactions. In short: a lot of suffering.

To find the "one" broken-down car, one that had lived long enough to be liberated from its "new car smell" but was still functioning well enough to not have gas leaks, fumes leaking, etc, was not easy. You can imagine the hunt ...

This time would be different. I was about to go on a car jubilee, to get a new car of my choice. I was about to buy a car that I actually would enjoy, one that I wanted.

## Living High in the Lord

I sniffed around, literally, and I came up with a car I liked, smell included. It was a beauty, a green Jeep Cherokee. I liked the idea of sitting high and was confident that the smells would be conquered, like everything else. I was a 110-pound woman, five feet four inches tall, and this was my first big car, one where I could sit up high. I loved this. I was having a heyday, sniffing new car fumes, sitting high above the other vehicles. I was living high in the victory; this was the healed life. I was in grace. All was well. I had a few great weeks … then, suddenly, I started to have symptoms!

## The Unexpected

The funny thing about land is, just when you think you know what is going on, just when you think you have it covered, something totally unexpected happens.

My foot, my small five-and-a-half size foot, eventually started experiencing terrible pain! My tiny tendons were irritated by driving a car that was much higher and larger than I was used to. My small foot could not extend itself properly or powerfully enough to reach the gas and brake pedals.

The distance between the seat and the pedals was a bigger stretch than I had realized. My foot was collapsing under the pressure. My new car was now three weeks old; I could not bring it back. I also could not drive it without terrible pain. My foot and ankle were swollen and sore. I looked at my options.

# Option One

I found a foot and ankle specialist. The doctor examined my weakened foot and ankle and diagnosed my condition as irritated tendons with a torn ligament. "This type of tear does often happen with smaller people in larger vans and trucks," he volunteered. "When the stretch is too great, it puts too much pressure on the tendons. It is not uncommon. I've seen it many times before."

I was amazed at how accurately he had aligned himself with the carnal mind's interpretation. *It must be some psychic thing doctors have,* I thought, *to hit you at your most vulnerable fear, almost demonic in insight.*

He continued. "All this has to be taken into consideration, and you must stay off that foot for at least three months for it to heal. No driving at all!"

The doctor prescribed physical therapy, pain medication, and rest. "Losing a car is better than losing a foot," was his parting remark.

I could no longer drive my car and now needed to go into physical therapy to repair the damage that I had done driving it this long. I would never drive my new car again! That was the medical point of view.

I was undaunted. Faithless physicians had long lost their sting; their intimidation process was almost encouraging at that point in my life! I decided against the physical therapy, which would take a year of ice, electrical stimulation, and exercises in a heated pool. You know the drill: lots of time, lots of money (probably the cost of two cars), lots of pain, interspersed with setbacks of despair. Then throw in the mental attack of confusion and the constant wondering and questioning of the impostor continuously asking, "Where is God?" Who on earth has escaped that torture?

## Tarrying

I threw out the prescription for pain pills, realizing that I would need to be as conscious as possible to take the land. Stoned land-taking was not an option! I further evaluated my situation and the medical suggestions. It was clear that I would be struggling with at least a year of disabled, victimized living. I knew that I could get healed faster than that. Why waste my time? My belief in my physical body as my identity had definitely changed. I wasn't buying it! Just biding time ... tarrying.

*Isaiah 40:31: "But they that wait upon the Lord, shall renew their strength; they shall mount up with wings like eagles; they shall run, and not be weary; and they shall walk, and not faint."*

## Temporary Plan

I called my spiritual sister, Linda; she volunteered to drive me around while my healing was coming to pass, till I figured out what was up. She would pick me up every day and we would do my day together. It was a lot of fun, but I didn't feel good about taking up her time and freedom.

I developed a temporary plan! I would get a car for the disabled — one for crippled people who couldn't use their legs or foot, and could be driven using just the arms. I would not have to stress the foot with the torn ligament and I would be able to drive, get around, and relax. Then, in peace, I would hear where the spirit of God was leading me ...

## The "Disabled" Car Mission

My friend Linda volunteered to pick me up. We went on a mission to rent a car that was for the disabled. What we didn't know was God already had His Plan. We felt that we were being righteous! After all, we were not sitting around complaining or waiting in the doctor's office as medical victims! I was not the recipient of physical therapy!

We were taking action. Wrong action is right action in the spirit. I am asked to step out, to press on to the mark for the high calling of God in Christ, to take action by faith. To be right is not necessary. I am not expected to be perfect. In healing, only faith is necessary. With the simple action of faith, God would begin to reveal, turn things around, and have an opportunity to move through somebody … If I step out in the wrong land, I am still righteous. I am in faith. Faith will create the miracle, not my "works." Grace is by faith. Grace is the supernatural miracle power of God.

It is sometimes difficult to "receive" grace when you are immobilized in fear. Just keep moving …

Linda and I drove out to the airport, having tracked down these precious, suitable vehicles. We made a reservation with a car rental place and had a distance to go to pick up the car. We were told that there would be a disabled-ready car waiting for us. It had begun to rain heavily in Los Angeles.

## First Stop: Who?

We arrived at the first car rental place and went into the office to get my reserved vehicle. They had never heard of me. They didn't have my reservation, and all the cars for the disabled had been rented, the last one just five minutes ago … "Next time, call."

## Moving On

We continued on our mission, called around, and were assured that there were many disabled-ready cars available. We went to the next city. We were driving all over the Los Angeles area. It had begun to rain harder, and the streets were flooding…

## Second Car Rental Place: Bad News!

We went on to the next place; they assured us on the telephone that they had an abundance of disabled-ready vehicles. We were certain this time; nothing could go wrong. We had tracked the cars down — they actually had forty of them. I only wanted one!

"Yes, we have many; you've come to the right place. Yes, we have your reservation. I need to see your license and I will have someone bring the car around back," the clerk assured us, taking my license and going off to do the necessary paperwork ...

## Doors Are Not Opening

We were waiting around for what seemed to be too long. Twenty minutes later, the clerk returned with bad news. "So sorry, we checked your license and found that it has been suspended due to a hit-and-run accident. Due to your driving record, we cannot rent you a car."

How embarrassing ... not true, but still embarrassing. We were beginning to get suspicious. We didn't mention it, not even to each other ... hmmm. We did notice that doors were not opening. Erroneous homicide-related accusations were not a good sign ...

## Third Car Rental Place

It was raining even harder now—torrential rains. We made another reservation, moving on. This time, we cleared my license with the clerk on the phone. We were prepared this time. I would get my car. Tomorrow, I would be a driver again!

A new problem emerged. My license was fine, but the two hundred disabled vehicles they had had yesterday — their entire fleet — had been moved to Orange County. It had just happened and they apologized. The employee who took the reservation was in the main office and had not been informed. Due to the rain, there was a delay in the fleet reaching its new destination. The records still showed that these vehicles were here in Los Angeles. My two hundred disabled-ready cars were floating somewhere in space — not available, untraceable, so sorry, blah, blah, blah … no car …

## Are You Getting This?

Our mission was becoming a comedy of errors. We walked out, stunned, and went back into Linda's car. She looked at me wide-eyed and said, "Are you getting this?"

We had not shared our thoughts to this point, not wanting to dampen the mission. "Yes, of course, I am getting this," I replied. We both laughed.

I felt it now; I had it now, just enough truth had been exchanged, agreed upon. There it was, God's plan, clear as day!

## The Cheech and Chong of Faith

"I got it," I shared with Linda. "I see it; it's over. I'm clear. I am not disabled. I am God's beloved daughter! I am the healed, redeemed, sanctified, and holy. Why on earth would I need a car for the disabled? What am I thinking? As far as the east is from the west am I, of all people, disabled!"

> Psalm 103:12: "As far as the east is from the west,
> so far hath he removed our transgressions from us."

We both laughed. We were hysterical now. How could we miss it? We both agreed how funny we were. We had been so certain! We imagined we were on prime time in heaven; spirits and angels had us on a big screen as entertainment. We were comedy in the spirit, the Cheech and Chong of faith!

We were amusing — driving around Los Angeles in the pouring rain seeking cars for the disabled. For a healed woman! I was free again. I had the answer. I was thinking clearly again. I was burdenless. We were traveling in a different mood. The atmosphere in the car had changed; we were in joy.

"Take me home," I said laughing. "I will get a car tomorrow. No problem—but not a car for the disabled, absolutely not. I will do the opposite: rent a car with a worse gas pedal position than my Jeep! I will have no trouble finding a truck, a big truck, one where I will hardly be able to put my foot down on the pedal."

## I Will Retaliate!

"Tomorrow," I said to Linda, "I will rent a huge, heavy diesel truck, with a gas pedal built for a giant. I will drive it to victory." We were gleefully laughing now. We felt it; we knew that it was righteous. There's a ring in the sound of truth, an elevation in its impartation. We had it; we knew it. We both had a peace about it.

## Not Giving It Up to a Gas Pedal

I was not about to give up my authority in Christ, my dominion, to a gas pedal! Not for a foot! Not for a million dollars ... Who I was and what I was doing had escaped me temporarily. I was back; it felt good. I was God's daughter, and all power had been given unto me. Thank you, Lord! I had experienced a temporary lapse in consciousness. That was the real problem. The foot thing could be easily resolved!

I would do what any spirit woman in Christ would do presented with such a circumstance. I would retaliate and gain power.

*2 Corinthians 12:9: "The power of Christ may rest upon me."*

## Led by the Spirit (God's Plan)

I woke up excited to conquer this new deception, and get my car and foot back. I had a new plan. I now had God's plan. I knew I was playing with a loaded deck.

My moving on in faith had created the redirecting revelation of the Lord. I had the trump card: Grace. *I had never suspected grace would be so hostile in its appropriation!*

## Got It, Lord!

I called a local car rental place, the closest and most convenient to my home. I inquired about a large diesel truck. No problem. There were many vans, trucks, etc. to choose from. They picked me up. No homicide suspicions, no cars mysteriously missing. They had what I needed: a yard full of heavy, ugly, diesel trucks — trucks that had gas pedals of lead. I walked out to the parking lot and tested different ones. I had never seen so many huge, ugly vehicles in my life! The pickings were good!

Then I saw my faith truck; it was perfect. I checked it out. I could hardly reach the pedal! The pedal itself was so heavy, it took all my strength to hold it down. I had to squat down to add a few pounds of weight to get enough leverage on the pedal to give the car enough gas to be able to move. I had the right one…

I had what I needed: an impossible truck. It required a stretch ten times worse than the original car that had allegedly torn my ligaments, and it had a gas pedal that was at least twenty times heavier!

## The Violent Take It by Force

Take a foot from me, hah! We'll see about that. I was a retaliator in action.

I was in God's will and power!

*Matthew 11:12: "The kingdom of heaven
suffereth violence, and the violent take it by force."*

The energy was strong; when it's God's plan, the energy is always strong. There was an edge in the atmosphere, a supernatural glory. Once the decision was made to step out, there was a pre-victory empowerment, a joy. Everything was going my way.

I was ready for the battle! It was about just walking it out. I had the revelation. I knew I was calling a battle that Jesus had already won. It was just about demonstrating my authority over this attack ... it would be a moment-to-moment battle. No one can know how to stand. It's a battle that is simply led, has many turns — a sensitive, primal, and violent battle.

The victory would be mine. The battle belonged to the Lord! The *"how to" belonged to the Lord. Vengeance is mine, sayeth the Lord (Romans 12:19),* and I was finding out that He was really good at it!

## The Action of Retaliation Faith

I was ready to go. I was tiny in my rental diesel truck, ridiculously small in it. I was certain that the rental agent was wondering what I was doing with a vehicle so inappropriate for my size. I was about to make my point or lose a foot.

## The Battle of the Foot

It was a beautiful Southern California day, sunny and bright, the air clear from yesterday's rain. I got in my truck; for me it was almost like mounting a horse. I climbed in, jumped up in it, and there I was ... sitting in the middle of this huge seat, looking more like a rag doll, a toy left behind, than a full-size driver! I proceeded to move forward, no particular place in mind, not unlike Moses in the desert; he knew that God would find a way! I knew that the Red Sea would part. How and when was the mystery of God! Faith just keeps moving ahead. I was taking a drive in an impossible vehicle. Impossible is the key word for a Battle of Retaliation.

## Impossible

Impossible means that I cannot, in my own power, accomplish this task. Impossible means that I have surrendered it totally to God. In my "impossible," I am making my position clear. I have surrendered. *I am in faith; I am busting a con, exposing a deception. I have upped the ante, and I am retaliating!*

## A Righteous Position

I was taking my righteous position as a healed woman, calling the bluff of deception. Whether you like to think this bluff is of the ego, the impostor, the mortal mind, carnal mind, or devils is irrelevant to your outcome! Do not allow how you see it, or name it, to disempower you from taking your right action.

*As long as you are upping the ante and calling the bluff of the con that is presenting evidence contrary to your divine health, authority and peace on this earth, you will have the victory.* If you desire to embrace your ego, inner self, inner child, etc, you will not be healed. You will be seduced into agreeing with your oppressor.

You must identify that this is not you at all; this is an imitation of you, a counterfeit, an impostor! There was an opinion going around that taking care of oneself is about being gentle, about nurturing oneself, perhaps taking a hot bath. My heart was not my inner child. My heart wanted a car. I wanted to drive! If I was the caretaker of my spirit, mind and body, I was going to have to guard my heart by setting it free, by eliminating a limitation. My heart and spirit wanted to get out of the nurturing bathtub and into life!

## The Truth Was

In my understanding, I was calling the bluff of my carnal mind, my old nature. I was in the war of the flesh and the spirit, and I had to bring my flesh under subjection … that was my job. I had inherited my authority as a child of God. I was redeemed from my old nature, translated by one blood offering, to be the righteousness of God in Christ. I was the regenerated spirit woman, the image and likeness of God.

That was my basic stand! It was my divine right to have a foot … I had to have a righteous indignation about it. I had to get there authentically. I had to feel it! I could feel the wrath of God.

Yes, God has wrath about deceptions. The battle was primitive and had great wisdom, simultaneously. This would not have been so easy for me to perceive years ago as a psychologist. I had spent years being the "inner child," a generational recipient of abuse and error — hardly the warrior of a living God.

*Galatians 5:17: "For the flesh lusteth against the Spirit, and the Spirit against the flesh: and these are contrary the one to the other: so that you cannot do the things that ye would."*

## I Will Drive to San Francisco

My next battle strategy was to simply turn on the truck's radio. I was beginning to enjoy a little music, cruising along. My foot was definitely feeling the pedal. It was such a powerful truck. My foot couldn't handle my much smaller Jeep; it couldn't handle a Ford Fiesta at this point! My foot was starting to go into serious pain. The opposition was attacking. I was listening, staying aware of my opponent's voice.

Listening is a very important part of the battle. *If you don't hear, you cannot retort properly. If you do not hear, you are not separate from your opponent.*

241

## A Toxic Babbler

My adversary began babbling fast, provoking fear. "You'll never walk again. You'll never drive again, and that is for sure! The doctor said you needed to stay off that foot. Are you crazy? You're not thinking clearly; you are out of your mind. This is a fantasy; you belong in therapy! This is not a disease; this is your foot. Your one and only right foot for life, and you are destroying it!"

The constant hostile onslaught of negative verbiage was accompanied by serious swelling and more pain! I continued driving, over the canyon hills now. I was leaving the city of Los Angeles and driving through the San Fernando Valley. I did not pull over or stop the car.

"I am healed," I retorted, still driving. "It is my right to be pain-free. This is a deception, and I will not buy it! I am a healed woman. You are a liar, a fake — a counterfeit!"

## The Battle Unfolds

I was hanging on to my spiritual reality. My foot was starting to look like a clubfoot; my ankle was swollen, enlarged and throbbing.

The impostor of my identity commented, "Look! Look at your foot! You are ruining your tendons and ligaments. All of them! Look at the swelling this driving is creating, and stop this! What are you trying to prove? This pain is not of God; you'll be crippled for life. You'll be in a vehicle for the disabled permanently. You're wrong this time. Get out; stop this car at once and call an ambulance. Get help!"

## Mental Idols (A Bluff)

Mental idols of doubt and fear were babbling faster than I was driving! They knew that it was now or never. All evil had were words and lying symptoms to justify its lies. As if my body had a mind, a life of its own! I refused to pull over!

Finally, I was practically unconscious with foot and ankle pain. My foot was throbbing. My opposition was screaming, "Stop this now! Stop this car! You are creating irreversible damage. Pull over and get out of this car! Look at that foot! Oh, my God!"

I continued to refuse to let go; more swelling and pain were imparted to me from that un-rebutted perception! The impostor wanted me to think that the pain was coming from driving the car! As if I was some victim without God in a material world! Powerless over my own flesh! Had my Lord not provided all I needed to be in the fullness of His authority on this earth?

## The Moment of Truth

There is a moment of truth in a spiritual battle, and we were upon it. To evaluate the outcome now, in the flesh, one would have to say that it didn't look good for me. My foot was swollen to twice its normal size. I was way above my pain threshold. The presented evidence was not in my favor.

I was not moved, because I could not be. I was not me anymore, not Juliana the human with foot pain, not the me that freaks out about pain. I had become the fullness of my spiritual self. I was giving place to my spiritual ideas, thoughts, identity and actions.

The warfare continued. I spoke a poignant truth: "I separate myself from you, totally. Your pain is not my pain, and I am not you. As far as the east is from the west am I from you. I am not my flesh. I am not my foot. I am not my ankle. I am on to your con. I know what you want! You want to immobilize me through my foot, keep me out of moving ahead in my life, and victimize me for months. With what? An illusion? A deception? What do you really have?"

243

I felt more power from these declarations. Not less pain, but more power! "I'm not pulling over," I continued. I then received more pain and more power.

Evil was reacting to my words. I went on. "My life is dead, I am hid in Christ. I am not pulling over; I am not getting out of this car."

Then suddenly, there it was, my helper; the Holy Spirit had arrived and was upon me, taking over. I was feeling the spirit of God now; glory was all over my car. The atmosphere was charged with a final battle edge. The devil had a bluff; the bluff was a threat with words ... mere words ... I had the action of faith (upping the ante).

The power of God is not just in words, but faith in action. I was in a demonstration of the finished work of the Cross of Calvary via retaliation faith. God would meet me here.

## If I Have to Drive to San Francisco

"Shut up," I continued. "I'll do the talking. Let me tell you something ... If I have to drive to San Francisco today, right now, I will. I will, and I am. (I had merged with the Holy Spirit; I was in the battle with inspired power now.) I don't care what you think or say, I am on my way. I will not stop this car; I will drive long and hard. I will keep driving ... I will not eat or sleep ... I will keep driving! I will not pull over. I will not rest. I will drive! All power has been given unto me, in heaven and on earth. (Matthew 28:18)

"I am not impressed with your lying symptoms. There is nothing you can do to get me to stop driving this car! I am separate from you; I am not you. This is my car, and I will drive it. This is my foot, and I will use it! You don't tell me what to do. I am your master. I totally separate myself from you. That's right, I am totally separate from you. I command my foot to be separate from your deceptions. My foot is not yours to manipulate! I am driving to San Francisco right now."

I said it, and I meant it with all my heart and all my soul. I put my car in the direction of the 101 Freeway and headed north.

I wasn't the one bluffing. I had real goods. I may have been calling a bluff, but my words were not idle threats (they were literal threats to the idol). I would back up every word with corresponding action!

My authenticity was communicated in the battle; everyone always knows exactly where everyone stands in a spiritual battle. I had the power now. I would not be backed down.

I felt Evil begin to slowly release its hold. I was acknowledged for who I am. All of a sudden, the enemy of my soul, health and wellbeing was thwarted, deflated. Evil realized that I was serious. "She knows, she knows who she is; she knows who He is. We had better back up."

## The Spirit Takes Over

"Back up," I began to speak with an inner authority. My voice had changed; it was louder, deeper, stronger. It was the voice of eternal power. It boomed in my innards!

"Back up; I've had it! I am going to San Francisco and that's it ... back up. You must back up all the way now. I will not be stopped. I will not be tossed by you. I shall not be moved by you." This debate was internal. I was not speaking outside myself. I made a quick left onto the freeway with a determination, a will, a force. I was on my way, going to San Francisco ...

I felt greatly energized by my own decision, my own declarations. My own words had increased my strength. I continued in the Holy Ghost. "I have had it. I am as Mt. Zion, which cannot be removed, but abideth forever.[28] This is it ... I shall not be moved![29] I shall not be moved![30] I separate myself from you."

---

28  Psalm 125:1
29  Psalm 16:8
30  Psalm 16:8

245

"I have set the Lord before me; He is at my right hand. I shall not be moved. I am totally separate from you! I am not you! For by one offering he hath perfected forever they that are sanctified.[31] Hallelujah! I am the sanctified. Yes, sanctified. I am separate from you, totally separated and in control of you. With the fullness of my authority in Christ, right here and right now, I am separate from you. You do not dictate to me what is going on in my body. I dictate what I want my body to do for me. My body belongs to me, not you. You are my slave, to obey me.

"I don't believe your words. You are a deceiver. I am not conned by them. It's my foot, healed by grace. Remove yourself and your lie from my body right now. I command you to release me now! Get thee hence, impostor!"

My action and my words complemented each other. The impostor was still attacking, but it was clear that I had the power. I drove my truck farther north on the 101 Freeway ... and pursued my righteous rebuttal.

I continued with spiritual enthusiasm and momentum. "You have no power over me. Your power doesn't come from above. There is no power but the power of God.[32] He is my rock and my salvation, and I shall not be moved.[33]

"I am on to you, I know what you want. I am not relinquishing my God-given authority over you. *This is not about my foot; get off my foot. This is about my identity, and you cannot take it.* I am rooted and grounded in Him. I am grafted into the vine.[34] My life is dead; I am hid in Christ.[35]

"I am going to San Francisco and you will not move me. You will not take my foot away on a con job. This I know, the foot of the righteousness shall not be moved.[36]

"Do not confuse yourself with me. I am not you. I am born of God; the seed of God, not of corruptible seed, but incorruptible, by the word of God, which liveth and abideth forever.[37]

---

31  Hebrews 10:14
32  Romans 13:1
33  Psalm 62:2
34  Romans 11:12

35  Colossians 3:3
36  Proverbs 12:3
37  1 Peter 1:23

"Now shut up! That is it!" I put my music on as loud as possible. "This conversation is over." I had stated my truth, declared my identity. I was going to San Francisco. I took my swollen foot and pressed it on the pedal as hard as I could. "I shall drive to San Francisco with my foot pressed down like this," I warned. My foot was spread out, fully and freely covering the gas pedal, holding nothing back.

## Bluff Called

That was it ... Glory to God in the Highest![38] Bluff called! My foot was healed in a flash. With that last threat of even further retaliation, my position was understood! Suddenly, the impostor took its hands (illusions) off my foot.

In a second, all the swelling went down, all the pain dissipated, my foot was back to normal. My opposition had bowed. I had backed the impostor up, and I was free! I turned my truck around and headed back towards Los Angeles. I drove peacefully, comfortably, back to the car rental place and returned my truck.

The whole process took one-and-a-half hours, not a year in physical therapy. No prayer line, sans therapy and no potential nervous breakdown over this new stress. No long discussions and months of confusion, playing the carnal mind control game of, "Lord, what should I do?"

I went home and drove my new toxic, smelly, green Jeep painlessly, with a stronger foot than the one I had had before this attack. My foot would no longer have any pain at all, ever again!

My foot had been strengthened in truth. I was no longer a passive vessel for foot and ankle pain. Never again. Conquered. This lie had had its last day of conning my mind and destroying my foot and ankle with deception. Another body part restored... Another idol mortified!

*Romans 8:13: "For if ye live after the flesh, ye shall die: but if ye through the Spirit do mortify the deeds of the body, ye shall live."*

38 Luke 2:14

# Chapter 37

## A Dance of Retaliation

I was never really out of back pain. I just had so many other, more pressing pains and issues that I could not devote my attention to it! I did get some back healing when I put the alleged toxic mercury back in my mouth. My back had felt better, but I would still throw it out every once in awhile.

The adversary had a story, and that story went like this: "You have had years of being weakened by lupus and environmental illness and this has taken its toll on your flexibility and structure."

With this deception hidden in my unconscious, I was a sitting duck for error to tempt me. I would be fine for a season, but then, if I moved too quickly, lifted something without help, once again my pelvis and hip area would feel displaced, weakened and twisted. Then I would be in constant pain! The chronic "can't lift even a tissue" routine would return from the past.

I had not yet enforced my grace in this area ... and I had just done some laundry ...

## Lifting Laundry

The belief of this deception, the con that I had been agreeing with up until this day, was simple. Many of you, I am sure, have heard it for yourself. It goes like this: "Lifting throws your back out!! Be careful when you lift! You cannot lift! You have serious back problems!"

This threatening thought was always accompanied by pain! Any light or even tiny item lifted would cause pain. There was always a story, something would always be created to trigger the whole deception to begin again! A simple move, accompanied by an un-rebutted thought, would aggravate my back. And then my life would be limited again, requiring rest, causing worry, trauma, immobility, days lost, months lost. "Don't do this, can't do that."

I would be a slave to my back, my flesh, my carnal mind and the law of sin and death once again controlling my life. Sin consciousness was condemning me, because it could, if I thought it was me and if I agreed with this unsanctified identification error ...

## Here We Go Again

I had just completed some laundry. I had randomly lifted my towels up and out of the washer to put them in the dryer. That did it. I didn't know how I would empty the dryer, for I was lying flat on my back on the living room floor in pain.

My carnal mind immediately went into its fear agenda. *Oh, no, oh, no, not again! Not this back pain. I will be in pain for months.*

I automatically tightened my back brace, as if that would hold my back in place and glue me together. I needed to be stabilized! I felt as if my pelvis was unhinged from my low back ... it was completely twisted. My flesh was freaking out in pain.

My lower back felt tremendous pressure, as if it were being pushed out of its socket! There was a feeling of kicking and pounding in the entire pelvis area, front and back. I started to pray, not knowing what to pray, feeling nothing but pain and fear from the thoughts that I had already received by the carnal mind's onslaught of deception! I tried to still my overtaken mind by praying in the spirit.

## Prayer Makes Me Worse!

I noticed, after about five minutes of praying in the spirit, that my pain was getting worse. My back was actually reacting negatively to my prayer! I was shocked!

I decided to pray more, so that I could watch this connection more closely. I was beginning to separate myself, allowing myself to be sanctified from this deception. I continued to pray in the spirit with more awareness. I wanted to hear my opponent's voice! I knew that if I could hear and identify these words that were creating my back pain, I would be able to stop receiving them.

I prayed and listened simultaneously. The more I prayed, the worse my back pain became! I was not moving my back; I was just praying. The reaction to my prayer was a larger dose of pain. Who was pushing this button? What in me hated prayer? I thought this to be a very positive and insightful sign. It witnessed to me the total spirituality of the problem. I was encouraged!

## A Con Exposed

I was no longer my body in pain. I was a spirit woman watching my lower back and pelvis be attacked by a spirit that did not like prayer. This changed everything, in a strange way. It gave me faith. I replied directly to the thoughts and corresponding symptoms. "Well, you don't like prayer! I am wearing a back brace. I am not moving around; no pulling, walking, lifting, twisting, and yet you are creating more pain! You are creating pain to oppose prayer!"

I began to bust the con, to let the devil know I was on to the game. I knew I had authority over these thoughts and their corresponding lying symptoms!

## The Appointed Time

I had stepped into a moment of God, an unplanned serendipity, an appointed time. My spirit knew that it was my moment! I automatically started stepping in, moving forward, moving ahead, taking territory. I continued to expose the lie. "You don't like prayer! I see you have a negative reaction to prayer!"

It thrilled me to make that connection! I knew that I was privy to an observation of grace. "You don't like my praying," I continued. I actually laughed. "In that case, I'll pray a little more. I'll pray without my back brace on!"

## The Good Fight of Retaliation

I was retaliating now. My innate discernment had taken over! I was in the battle. All power would be given unto me. I was confident. "Why should I wear a back brace?" I said. "There is nothing wrong with my back! It is you causing my pain. My back has nothing to do with this! Absolutely nothing! No more back brace, that's it! I will not condone your antics!" I removed my back brace and flung it across the living room floor.

I continued to pray. I received more lying symptoms, more pain. "I see, devil, that you are responding to me. The tables have turned here! I am no longer sitting around passively, hoping to be able to do a little laundry!"

I began praying harder just to provoke and irritate the enemy of my soul! Fervent prayer in the spirit.[39] The effectual fervent prayer of a righteous man availeth much."[40] I taunted the devil, once again letting the enemy know that I knew who I was!

"You don't like my spirit praying," I mocked evil. "Good! You have blown your cover! I will pray even more!"

I was finally out of the back brace, feeling almost naked walking around my living room without it holding me together. I was in faith; my action of throwing off the back brace had led me out my immobilized spot! One step of faith had taken me straight to my position of righteousness! I began to express myself, empowered in spirit and truth! I moved on, walking,

39 Ephesians 6:18
40 James 5:16

251

strolling without my brace—making a grand show of my gained territory.

I was expanding my new turf, setting larger boundaries, taking land! I became walking prayer; my back was no better and no worse. I had to add a little Holy Spirit power!

## Adding Power

It was time to up the ante! I walked sans brace to my closet and picked out a pair of shoes. I had not been able to wear high heels for eight years. The amazing thing was I still carried them around! I put them on. I let the impostor know what I was taking.

My turn to intimidate! "You don't like prayer," I commented. "How about high heels? How about five-inch high heels? How do you like high heels, devil? How about dancing? How do you feel about dancing? How would you like to dance with five-inch high heels on? How would you like to be a dance of prayer, be a living worship?"

Previous to this battle, wearing a pair of high heels would have created a pain that would start in my low back and go all the way down both my legs, inflame my hamstrings, and totally cripple and disable me for months. It was out of the question to attempt to wear them without serious repercussions!

## Busting the Con

I was busting the con in the moment of God! I would add more faith to my warfare arsenal by taking back more than the devil was trying to take from me. I would take back what error had deprived me of for years. A clean sweep! I went to the stereo, chose a great dance CD. I chose one with wild and powerful dance music from the movie "Desperado."

I moved on to the prayer dance worship. I intended to give my opposition a little retaliation. I would tax the devil. Take a little extra.

# I Retaliate

I began dancing in my five-inch heels, no back brace, no protection. Evil was enraged, losing its cool, throwing random pains here and there, making no sense, just attacking and defending its lie!

In a warped way, it was blowing its own cover over and over! I had pushed its buttons — provoked it! I had triggered it! It was obvious it was busted; I had called it out!

The Lord had set a banquet before me in the presence of my enemies.[41] It was my battlefield now. I was no longer the unsuspecting generational victim of deceit whom it had hoped to take out for a few months. I had grown in faith.

# In the Spirit of Dance

I began dancing wildly through the pain, dancing bigger, harder, stronger, faster, freer, dancing in the spirit! I had not planned for this war; it was an unexpected battle. God had swung a door open, and I was going to walk (dance) through it!

I was dancing in opportunity, jumping up and down, demonstrating my authority over my body. I was doing things that I had not been able to do in years … I danced and danced. I turned, I twisted, I perspired. I was free in my movements, holding nothing back from my Lord.

It's amazing to me how the opposition enjoys taking away what you love — your heart's joys. I was taking it back. I danced on and on. I felt as if time had stopped. A holy moment was transpiring; it was God's timing. The dispensation of grace! (Ephesians 3:2)

I remembered, in this sacred space, my passion for dance. I danced with Jesus through weird pains, sitting in heavenly places. I had become the privileged observer of seeing evil throw

---

41 Psalm 23:5

deceptions through my mind, watching it trying to get me to submit to thoughts that were not true! If I agreed with the thought, I would receive the pain!

In my new upheld position, I was able to see clearly how these thoughts were coming in! I was astonished, amazed and humbled that I had allowed this oppression for all these years! I was being fortified by simply stepping out of my carnal identity and choosing to retaliate.

I was supernaturally placed above the thoughts of the flesh and became a separated overseer of these deceptions! I had just been translated — from being a receiver of an evil con job, a victim unable to see the thoughts of my deceiver, rendered unconscious by this deception — to being the aggressor in the battle. I liked it!

I kept dancing till I had moved all the unmovable parts of my body, till I twisted my pelvis around as if I were a belly dancer, as if it were a pretzel. Because I could. Because it was all a lie.

All these years, I had suffered in vain! I saw it now. A total deception! I would twist my pelvis if I wanted to twist it. I would lift when I wanted to lift. Who was this devil to tell me what to do, to dictate to me? I was rapidly becoming indignant, seeing this attack for what it was, for what it had been, years of suffering for naught, for a carnal story. Crippled over a false tale.

I was angry—a Holy anger. I was calling this carnal bluff with new vigor. I had bought this con; I had given my back and pelvis and my dancing over to a mere carnal mind control con.

My opponent was not silent. My opponent was talking trash; after all, talk is what it had, words were the game. Whose words would have the final say? Whose words would stand? Whose words would bow? Mine or sin consciousness?

Evil was warring with me for position, to steal my healing, my grace. Who would be left speaking, reigning? "You are destroying your back," it raged, throwing its favorite threat, the pain now all the way down the leg! Then a fresh tirade of pain followed this hostile and aggressive accusation — pain down my buttocks, and all the way down the back of my thighs to the back of the knees!

I was no stranger to the sacroiliac threat, "the one that takes months to get over," evil reminded me, "months of recovery. You'll never dance again or walk again!" it was screaming in defense of its position.

"You will have to lie flat in traction for at least six months to get over this damage that you are creating." As it spoke this malicious comment, the spirit of self-justification threw another pain, directed straight to the lower back.

My entire lower back area was feeling constricted. It felt like I was being cut in half, a demonic pull, as if there were a tight band pulling at my lower back. The carnal mind's thoughts would keep telling me over and over that I was destroying my back and then throw its corresponding pain to validate its remarks.

## Justified by Faith

"I'm justified by faith,"[42] I declared. "Shut up! I'm on to you; it's over. You are nothing but a scam, an illusion from hell!" That said, I danced faster, bigger, stronger, more. I sweated, I shook, I jumped, I rocked as the Holy Spirit instructed me: "Keep moving, just keep dancing. Deception is grasping at straws!"

"How will you survive without a back?" the oppressor declared. "Who will take care of you? Who do you think you are?"

"Wrong question, devil." I was enraged; the wrath of a living God encouraged me. "Who do you think I am, devil?" I replied.

42  Romans 5:1

"You know who I am, don't you? I am a vessel of the most high.[43] I am the new creature in Christ,[44] called with a holy calling,[45] taking nothing for myself and taking nothing from you.[46] Get thee hence, Satan.[47] Get thee hence!"

I was kicking now; I was in a spiritual kickboxing match, kicking the devil's butt! I, who could not lift a leg up higher than my own knee fifteen minutes ago, was violently kickboxing. My opponent had underestimated my righteousness.

"Who am I, devil?" my Godly wrath continued. "Who am I? All power has been given unto me in heaven and on earth.[48] I have inherited the fullness of the power of God,[49] the free gift of grace.[50] I have been given dominion on this earth![51] Dominion over you and all of your antics of evil![52] I am on to you! By one blood offering,[53] I am above all principality and power might and dominion.[54] I am a quickened spirit.[55] I am the seed of Jehovah,[56] El Shaddai. The Great I Am,[57] the only living God![58] I am redeemed from your authority and your law.[59] I am in the Perfect Law of Liberty,[60] hid in Christ.[61] Hallelujah! I am here to take you down. How dare you attack my back? You will pay for this attack! If I were you, I would back up now. Back up, Satan. Come under the subjection of the will of the Only Living God.[62] The only Eternal Immortal God;[63] The Great I Am, the Rose of Sharon, the Alpha and Omega, the beginning and the end.[64]

43 Psalm 82:6
44 2 Corinthians 5:17
45 2 Timothy 1:9
46 Matthew 6:25
47 Matthew 4:10
48 Matthew 28:18
49 John 1:12
50 Romans 5:15
51 Genesis 1:26
52 Romans 6:14
53 Hebrews 10:14
54 Ephesians 1:21
55 1 Peter 3:18
56 Galatians 3:29
57 Exodus 3:14
58 Jeremiah 10:10; Romans 9:26
59 Galatians 3:13
60 James 1:25
61 Colossians 3:3
62 Romans 13:1
63 Deuteronomy 33:27
64 Revelation 1:8

Bow, devil; you lost this battle two thousand years ago at the Cross of Calvary.[65] Bow to the Lordship of Jesus Christ![66] You have no choice. Bow!"

## The Victory Was Mine, the Battle ... the Lord's (1 Samuel 17:47)

I had it. I knew it. I felt it. I was possessing land; my essence knew what to do, led by the spirit of God. I was on fire from head to toe. The spirit of God had encapsulated me.

I loved the fact that I was dancing to "Desperado" and not praise music. God had led me to "Desperado," a wild and free tune, to not allow my enemy "sin consciousness" to pull any pranks or make this a one-time religious experience and undermine my authority. I was not going to allow the "law" to diminish what God was teaching me in the school of the spirit. That type of setup could be used later to take my healing back, with the impostor attempting to convince me that it was due to the praise music!

"No, I am on to you! I'll tell you what it is, devil. It is my dancing by faith in five-inch heels to 'Desperado,' swinging my pelvis, my lower back, my hips, stretching my hamstrings—dancing and prancing as a wild woman in the night. I want to remind you who I am, devil," I continued my verbal assault.

"My life is dead, and I am my authority in Christ, devil,[67] (Colossians 3:3) I am His righteousness:[68] that is my identity. I am a radically alive vessel of the Most High! I am the divine seed in action![69] Who are you? The law of sin and death,[70] the father of all lies,[71] a generational error from the beginning of time. You are nothing — a counterfeit of my identity. You are

65 John 19:17
66 Philippians 2:10
67 Colossians 3:3
68 Hebrews 11:7
69 Galatians 3:29
70 Romans 8:2
71 John 8:44

257

pretending to be me! You are a fraud, a bully, a con, an impostor! You are, in fact, under my feet, with which I will continue to dance!

"You have made a mistake, devil. If I were you, I would stop these hostile advances on my spirit. I will never give up my dance again. Not to you, not for anything. Never! I will dance when I want to dance. I will dance all night. I will take more territory."

I continued to dance; I had spoken my last retort. I was busy enjoying my dance. My point was made. The music was joining me in a crescendo. Antonio Banderas was having his victory in the movie at the same time. I was dancing; dancing in five-inch heels. I had the flesh under subjection. I had done my job. I had mortified the deeds of the flesh.

*Romans 8:13: "For if ye live after the flesh, ye shall die: but if ye through the Spirit do mortify the deeds of the body, ye shall live."*

## Knocking on My Door

All of a sudden, the battle was over. I had not planned for this warfare. This one had taken me by surprise. It had such shock value, I forgot that my friend Linda was coming over to do laundry, to help me move the clothes from the washer to the dryer. Suddenly, I became aware of a knock at the door. I had danced for more than forty-five minutes.

"How long have you been knocking, Linda?"

"About ten minutes," Linda said. "What is going on in there? I felt the spirit of God; the fire of God is in your house, all over your house. I felt it from the outside. The anointing of God is all over you," she exclaimed. "What is going on? What has happened? Who got healed? Who is in your house?"

"I retaliated for the attack on my back," I said. "God healed my back. All I can feel is the fire of God! God healed my back. There was so much fear, warfare and excitement that I can't feel anything. I can't even feel the joy right now. I know one thing. My back is healed! I can even wear heels. Look!" I threw my leg up in the air and freely displayed my five-inch high heel.

"Let's do laundry in heels," I added. "I can lift my own wet towels and anything else! I have no back pain."

## Round Two

I went to sleep that evening with great confidence and joy. I woke up with back pain — not as bad as it was after the laundry lifting, but not gone. My carnal mind took this opportunity to take me out. It was assuming that my stand was shaky, knowing that we mortals are weak in the morning, with the unconsciousness of the old creature still close to the surface.

Evil was trying to make a comeback! The old nature, manipulated by sin consciousness, started to work me over bright and early with its concepts, its lying words ready to undermine. "You accomplished nothing," it declared. "You haven't even left the bed yet, and you are still in pain!"

With that remark received — not rebuked, not rebutted — my whole back tensed. I was definitely feeling pain; the pressure in my lower back had returned. I had no reply.

It took that opportunity, that stall of my righteousness, to rapidly retort. Self-justification rambled on. "You can't move. You're still in pain; you'll probably get worse as you start to move around, as the day goes on. Not to mention the damage that has no doubt occurred from your "Desperado" dancing. That was just a temporary healing, just for that moment. You felt relief in your hysteria. This back problem of yours is not new. You have had this for fifteen years; it does not get healed in a moment!

"If it were truly healed, you would not have pain again today! You had better get up, if you can, and examine what's left of your back."

With that remark delivered, I received a corresponding tension along with additional tightness and more pain, this time delegated to the hip area, the old pelvic twist. I lay there stunned, gathering my thoughts, my reality.

The hostile and aggressive remarks had drained me. The words of my enemy created an energetic vacuum. I felt weakened from head to toe.

Temptation went on. "You were in some hyper trance state, dancing last night. This is the light of day."

This time I got a pain right to the coccyx; at the tip of my pelvis, an immediate inflammation occurred.

"You have fibromyalgia and arthritis," self-justification reminded me, taking a medical shot. "The x-ray was clear. Do you think you can dance fibromyalgia away? Why isn't everyone with fibromyalgia out dancing, then?"

More inflammation, more fear, and then my head began to throb, an extra bonus of fear.

"Put that back brace back on. You'll feel better. You probably are a little better; you were terrible yesterday. At least today you can walk. Be grateful for what you have today. Relax, no physical activity. Take an aspirin for your headache, and go back to sleep. If you exert your body today, you will do irreversible harm."

## A Spiritual Alzheimer's

I had a decision to make. I could be intimidated into relinquishing my power. I knew that my identity was what the opposition was after. If I forgot who I was, I would believe this voice to be my voice. It would be an unconscious bow, a bow without battle, just a total stripping of my power. A spiritual Alzheimer's. It would be a total forgetting of my life, my purpose, and my destiny, an utter disregard of all that I am.

The enmity of God would like me to become a blank recipient of lies, deceptions, and cons predetermined from the beginning of time. To be quite honest, I was a little spaced out. I had been hit in the battle. I had lost my expression.

I knew one thing. Lying there and listening to this rhetoric was the very worst thing I could do. I had to find strength to move, to get up. I had to find my will. Knowing what I had to do, identifying it, helped. It was a conversation on my side, acknowledgment coming from my spirit.

## More Action, More Power

I got out of bed; I was taking action. I walked in terrible pain, but I walked. "I am not putting my back brace back on," I said. "No way. I am not; let's get that straight. I am not putting my back brace on. No matter what happens, the brace stays off!" I had had a taste of back freedom, and I was not giving it up!

I knew that, in this moment, I had heard too much. I did not have rebuttal power, to push it back with words. I would have to put a little faith in this battle, get a little of God's power. God's power would come by faith, the action of faith.

"This is a grace war, after all, devil," I declared. "Not a debate! I will demonstrate who I am." Instead of putting my back brace on, I put my five-inch high heels back on. I would do another round of 'Desperado.'

## More Dancing

I danced through another forty-five minutes of battle; I danced through the lies, through the pain, through the threats, and again I had the victory. All power had been given unto me … (Matthew 28:18) I did this every day for four consecutive days. Each morning, I would wake up with pain, less than the day before, and each day, I would confront my oppressor by faith. By the fifth day it was over. I woke up in total freedom. I had backed the back attack down … forever.

## The Impostor Wants You Down

The old nature, beloved, will always try to take your healing back. The carnal mind will use any line of thinking that you may be personally susceptible to, taken straight from the bank of your generational seed principality — the inherited conditions of your parents, their parents, back through your entire bloodline to the beginning of time. It might sound like this: "You can't dance. Your mom never danced because of her disabling back pain. Bad backs run in your family. Your dad had a sacroiliac dysfunction. Grandma had a pelvic problem all her life—you remember, she was on pain medication."

## Cons to Recognize

Another common deception con is: "You have had back pain all your life because of your situation. After all, you have been injured! You were in an accident. That really happened!"

That remark would, of course, be followed by additional self-justification validation. "Doctor so-and-so diagnosed it as a blah, blah." And so it goes. The enmity of your wellbeing enjoys using a medical or psychological diagnosis to validate and justify itself.

## Unholy Book of the Law

These misinterpretations of your identity and spiritual status are the scriptures of error, the Unholy Book of the law's doubt and condemnation. No matter how your situation came about, you are not controlled by your body. You have authority, dominion over it; you are the master of your flesh. Your body is representing the thoughts of your opposition, the carnal mind. I assure you that disharmony and pain are all deceptions trying to call your bluff. Turn on it! Do not be conned! Identify deception, call its bluff, bust the con, up the ante, and praise the Lord! Hallelujah!

# Chapter 38

## Additional Retaliations

I believe that there is enough faith in these testimonies themselves to prepare one to receive the revelation for one's own personal retaliations, and empowerment therein. The regenerated spirit quite naturally responds to and is inspired by truth. We are healed by the blood of the Lamb and the word of our testimony. (Revelation 12:11) Following are more real life testimonies of bringing the flesh under subjection with proper spiritual identification and the authority of Jesus Christ ...

Here is another simple story of a demonstration of the battle between the flesh and the spirit, applying Divine Retaliation faith principles.

## Don't Settle for Less

I was involved in a minor automobile collision. I was not injured badly. My knee, however, did hit the dashboard and was swollen and blue. This did not concern me much after all the healing and victory I had experienced with my body. A simple knee inflammation was not going to create that much anxiety. I walked every day and I had no intention of giving up my walking or anything else!

## I Walk by Faith

The next morning, I awakened not taking much thought about the whole situation. I had made a decision of faith. "I am not giving up my walk." I stated my position internally to put the old nature on notice.

"I will walk this day and God will meet me and my knee will be healed!"

"Your knee has turned blue overnight and is very swollen," was the retort of my adversary.

I began my walk. I was walking, or trying to walk, but my knee was crumbling in pain. My knee was not going along with my plan. Of course, my knee is not an individual; it is just flesh. It has no personal consciousness!

Everything my knee feels is a command coming from a thought, either an unconscious thought, a carnal thought of sabotage, or an enlightened thought of the spirit. The body does not have a personal mind. It is not a master; it is a slave. I think Bob Dylan said it well: "Everybody has to serve somebody sometime, either the devil or the Lord."

I did not allow this fleshy deception to arrest my walking. I let my knee, and my carnal mind, know once again, "I will not give up my walk." I repeated my intent. "I will *not* relinquish my walk!"

What I thought would be a simple stand was turning into a greater challenge! I was declaring that I was walking, but my knee continued to buckle. Perhaps by now the reader is suspecting what I was not yet seeing. If you are getting what I was not seeing, you are ready to do some serious retaliating. I continued to walk. I knew that I could not give my walk up. We all know by now that I am not going to be relinquishing my walk!

A verbal battle unfolded. I said, "I am walking."

The opposition laughed. "You are not walking; you are falling down."

This was a fact; I was saying that I was walking, but with every step I attempted to take, my knee was buckling and I could not hold myself upright. I would fall. Then I would pick myself back up and we would start all over again.

"I will not give up my walk," I declared with great faith.

"Ha! Ha! Ha!" evil grunted. "You are not walking."

Boom, down I went again, with my knee again buckling under me.

I began listening more closely to the internal voice of my opposition, wanting to get the impostor's line of thinking so that I could give a proper rebuttal. "I have all authority over you," I continued. "You will do as I say. If I say walk, I walk." I began to walk and, once more, I was thrown to the ground, in the dirt, my battered knee already wounded, scraped, bleeding, and now filthy like the rest of me!

It was a hot summer day. I was wearing shorts and my knees, legs and hands were now full of mud! I was not a victorious sight. I picked myself up, wiped myself off and began to walk again. I was totally focused on this battle, and with all of my strength I was trying to hold my knee up, to keep my legs in a walking position, but I kept falling down.

The impostor of my identity was ecstatic! Evil was triumphing and starting to go into a demonic chant. "You can't walk; you can't walk. You say that you are walking, but you are not walking. You can't walk. You are seriously injured from the accident. You are not healed; you cannot walk. You are falling down."

"I can walk; I will not relinquish my walk. I am a healed woman, by my position of righteousness, by the blood of Jesus, by His grace, by His word. I can walk," I responded, and then my knee crumbled and I was on the floor again, dirty, in pain, not walking. Obviously, I was not walking. Talking, but not walking!

## You're Right, I Can't Walk

I may not have been walking, this is true, but I was in the land. I was in faith, and I was in God's Plan. I was not in my head, deliberating. I was in action. I was in God's will. This would give me favor. I knew this. However, I was not yet able to walk.

## Not Walking

I tried once more to get up to walk; I got knocked down. "That's not walking," evil noticed. "That is you falling down. You are an idiot," it accused. "No walking involved in your walk today. Go home. You are wasting your time. Go home, lie down, and let that knee heal. Put some ice on it. You are probably infecting it now. All this dirt on an open wound is not good. Go home. It is not of God for your knee to get infected. You can try again tomorrow."

The voice of evil was trying to get me to drop my stand and lose a little power, replace my faith with fear, then have me bow to it … and add an idol. I found myself thinking in truth …

> *Romans 8:15: "For ye have not received the spirit*
> *of bondage again to fear; but ye have received*
> *the Spirit of adoption, whereby we cry, Abba, Father."*

After that spiritual idea, I had a realization. This ungodly manifestation of rebellion would love to have an opportunity to swell my knee up overnight and put the inflammatory emotion of fear on it while I slept. Evil wanted to seduce me into passivity and then convince me into receiving additional lying symptoms!

## Give No Place to Deception

It is not good to give up a day—an hour—even a moment to deception. Giving up a day could become giving up a week; giving up a walk, a leg. Why walk around in the curse? I was holding fast to the liberty in which Christ had set me free. Not entangled again with the yoke of bondage. (Galatians 5:1)

## I Will Not Walk (Another Round)

"I will walk," I declare. "I will walk." Then, as I sat recovering from another toss in the dirt, I "got" it. I had the revelation. I got back up once again, laughing this time. I was, after all, in the land, and by that step of faith I had positioned myself for the *redirective revelation*!

"You're right," I said. "You're absolutely correct. I cannot walk. Ha! Ha! I will not try to walk again, not today. There will be no walking today. Absolutely no more walking today!"

The Lord had flashed through my heart the understanding; the simplicity of the primal battle that I was in ... I then knew what to do. I had been trying to fight the impostor on its chosen territory: "the walk."

I had to up the ante! Tax the devil a little bit. Take a little extra! Get larger than the attack. Demonstrate my dominion!

"Today, I run!" I flew up like an athlete, as an eagle in the Lord. No problem now. I took off and finished my walk by running and jogging. My knee, of course, was totally healed!

> Isaiah 40:31: "They that wait upon the Lord shall renew their strength; they shall rise up with wings of an eagle; they shall run, and not be weary, and they shall walk, and not faint."

# Chapter 39

## Spiritual Craftiness

I had to set my stakes a little bit higher; I upped the ante on deception and busted the con. Bust the con, up the ante, and praise the Lord! Divine Retaliation always gets on the bigger horse and shows its power. The regenerated spirit, all-knowing, never attempts to fight the devil on the adversary's chosen territory! The spirit is too crafty for that.

The mind of Christ is an eternal, immortal mind. Why should I fight for just what is being taken from me, why spend my life holding on to what I have? That's a losing battle, a retro battle. I would be deceived into looking back! Why should all my time be spent hanging on to my body parts? I am His righteousness, all His power is mine, all power has been given unto me... I am God's beloved Daughter.

I cry Abba, Father (Romans 8:15) and King of Heaven and Earth is my backup!

Faith is not about trying to save my butt or my knee and then having me feel good about it, as if I have been healed of something great! No, I already had a knee; the knee and my daily walk in peace were already mine. I was trying to win the battle without fully accepting my dominion.

I was contaminating my faith by holding back my true primal instincts, the fullness of who I am. My position in Christ is always the same! No matter how I feel, how I look, how the situation looks, my authority on this earth is secured by the blood of Jesus. *If I am willing to negotiate this fact, I am allowing my identity to be undermined, and the impostor will not budge. Evil will call my bluff.*

When I up the ante, and show the impostor that I am fully aware of the blood of Jesus and my rights therein, the impostor must bow to me. Deception must bow to faith and truth. There is no contest. This is not a guessing game. It is an absolute fact. The Lord Jesus Christ has won this battle.

*Hebrews 5:14: "How much more shall the blood of Christ, who through the eternal Spirit offered himself without spot to God, purge your conscience from dead works to serve the living God?"*

The curse of the law has been broken; its hold was paid for! The law has no power over you! The Cross of Christ was not suffered in vain. If the Cross of Christ was truly accomplished, you might ask, why is there still suffering and victimization amongst believers?

There is an answer, beloved ...

## The Law Is Faking It!

The law is faking it! That is all. The law is faking its authority over you! It's a con job! Don't settle for less; it can cost you a battle! You could be led by error to believe that God is not meeting you!

You may be asking for too little.

Asking for less is the counterfeit's deception to keep you out of victory! Go for what you really want! Take back the fullness of what was taken from you and add the impossible. Add the dream. Tax, tax, tax the devil!

Don't get small in retrieving your dominion. Get righteously indignant! You are righteously indignant; you just may not be feeling it yet! The law will attempt to numb your heart in oppression with unidentified words of subtle condemnation and disempowerment. These thoughts, if received, will repress your true feeling of holy anger at this sin consciousness scam. You will feel depressed at being overtaken.

Grief is the emotional smokescreen for the carnal mind. You are being led by deception—no more, no less.

This carnal grief, straight from the law, is nothing more than a distraction, a ploy to take your focus off of what you have to do. Depressed people do not retaliate. They are jammed in condemnation, rendered useless in the battle, kept on the sideline, not up at bat, no home runs, no opportunities, sitting life out on the bench.

The law wants you thinking, agreeing with, and abiding in the mind of carnality. Once you are there, you are more receptive to the next sequence of sabotage, which will inevitably be "the impostor inquisition." It jams your mind with worthless questions, as you try to figure out what happened to you. Wondering, planning … Evil knows that there is no faith in your pondering. No faith, no grace. Grace is by faith. (Ephesians 2:8)

## The Identity Attack

When you are attacked, the opposition wants you to submit your identity in Christ. The identity thief (the impostor) will try to keep you out of the only real battle! That battle is for your identification, which has been secured by the blood of Jesus.

> James1:17 "Every good and perfect gift is from
> above, and cometh down from the Father of lights,
> with whom is no variableness, neither shadow of turning."

Your position of righteousness in Christ is stable, and in it, you did not err. You absolutely did not create the error you are in! I am not talking about not taking responsibility for your actions. I am talking about a deception that will keep you in works all your livelong days — a deception that wants to justify its behavior by condemning you.

I am talking about a deception that wars with you for your grace! A constant and perpetual enemy that has you, its very master, seeking healing from "it." Your "inner terrorist" (the off-spring of the law) knows that you have the power of God over it. This enmity wants you convinced that there is something wrong with you! You need to be fixed! It wants to heal you, change you, cunningly trying to create a stumbling block to your grace!

## Done Deal

I assure you, beloved, that your translation is complete, done! You are healed, transformed, delivered, hid in Christ. You are piggybacking on an accomplished victory over the law. The law is your last and final stand. We no longer need to fight for what is ours, to seek outside medical or psychological assistance for the gifts and grace of God.

All that self-help seeking is the self-righteousness of the law trying to seduce you into the systems of the world. This entire ploy is a plot to steal your position of righteousness and trap you into the stumbling block of works. If you are seduced into "self-help," you can fall from your grace and ultimately be victimized.

*Romans 8:2: "For the law of the spirit of life in Christ Jesus hath made me free from the law of sin and death."*

## One Rule

By keeping the simplicity that is within Christ vibrant, we understand the only real problem. Only one thing can go wrong; you were misled. If you have a bad situation, a problem, an accident, etc. ... you were not led by God! Evil deceived you and misled you, hoping aggressively to blame and trap you, to condemn you! That's what happened ... One problem, one solution!

271

The Lord has provided for your training and perfection in being led. You are forgiven! When you are misled, you are forgiven, and you receive immediate grace to pick yourself up, brush yourself off, and get redirected in the spirit. This new leading will straighten out the old problem.

It is a natural law of grace. You may walk freely into the new "next" moment of God. That is your best defense. *This action of faith in the new moment will activate your grace.* Then let go; don't look back or think back. Move on and be supernaturally blessed.

## The Impostor Inquisition Uses Doubt

The only thing that can stand between the immediate re-leading and your immediate blessing is getting jammed, {stuck} in your head. This is done with the temptation of questioning. It can sound like this:

> "What went wrong? What should I do? I should have done this. I should have done that. What can I do now? What is the will of God in this situation?"

These kinds of thoughts are the deceiver's allies. Identify them and move on. They are simply kicking you when you are down. This is dirty fighting. Tell it to shut up. It is just trying to get you into doubt and condemnation. Tell it plainly and loudly that this is your bottom line: "There is therefore now no condemnation in Christ" (Romans 8:1) and keep moving.

Choose an anti-condemnation scripture to become your all-inclusive stand, a final word that will have power over all. "There is therefore now, devil, here and now—this minute, in my life, in my body, in my heart, in my mind, in my bones, in my thoughts, in my words; there is, therefore, now no condemnation in Christ. His grace is sufficient; my sins are forgiven. So shut up."

## Tax and Train

Then tax the devil a little. Train evil to obey you by retaliating.

When attacked with the "intellectual impostor," let go of everything, and enjoy your day. Take a few hours off from all responsibilities. Just let go of all concerns and focus on what evil hates above all things — a good time. *By the next day or in a few hours, by your action of faith, you will remember who you are and know what you have to do. Let go. Cast your cares on Him; He will work it out. (1 Peter 5:7)*

## Simply Switch Sides

Everything you need has been provided for you at the Cross of Calvary. Switch sides! Turn on these lies with the wrath of God (Romans 1:18). God is not teaching you via condemnation.

The Lord has delivered you from all guilt and condemnation! That is what the Cross of Calvary was about!

The Lord took the law of sin and death and every curse it could create and annihilated it. He has separated you from the generational victimization of your ancestors.

## Call a Battle

If there is a place in your life where you are continually attacked, feeling bad, joyless or suffering, *instead of trying to eliminate it or do better next time: call a battle!* Stop working it out in the natural realm.

Retaliate, and God will lift you up! I am saying that you cannot do it better, faster, or in a more enlightened manner than simply fighting one solo primal battle: "The Grace War." The war of retaliation. You just simply cannot!

The evil one will create ongoing battlefields for you if you decide to become an ambitious Christian in the law … a religious Christian. A believer deceived into being carnal and not spiritual is a believer suffering in vain with illness and confusion.

273

This is a believer with all power over his or her situation who is just not aware of His all-encompassing grace ... Spirituality is where your power is.

One battle, one mind, one Lord. (1 Corinthians 8:6 or Ephesians 4:5) ... in Christ ...

## Vessel Job Description

My job is to recognize my inheritance in every circumstance, understand it, agree with it, praise God for it, and enforce it! I enforce my grace by the action of my faith. I demonstrate my dominion by bringing my flesh — and, with it, the generational principality behind it and its master, the law of sin and death — under subjection!

I am, after all, His righteousness. What else would I possibly do? I no longer have to learn and grow via the punishment of condemnation and guilt! I cannot sin; I am spirit! If I am accused of compromise, I must enforce my identity and retaliate. This creates further sanctification, more detachment from the thoughts and temptations of the counterfeit, and a greater ability to perceive the con job. If I am deceived (misled) by error, I am promoted! I go to the lessons of life in the joy of the Lord.

> Hebrews 9:12: "By His own blood he entered in once into the holy place, having obtained eternal redemption for us."

## The Voice of Faith

Faith says, "Take something from me, and you will dearly pay. It will cost you. Take something from me, and you will lose. I am your master. I will teach you and train you to obey me, to come under the subjection of the will of God."

> 1 Corinthians 9:27: "I keep under my body, and bring it into subjection."

## Faith Sees Truth

"I give commands, and you bow," that's how faith sees it. "I am the head and not the tail," that's how faith sees it. Faith perceives its total authority over evil, its total separation, its sanctification, one mind, one life in Christ! Faith demonstrates its spiritual truth. The spirit person enjoys taking its rightful place. You will only be satisfied and happy when you are in God's will and purpose. No one will disagree with me there. You will be attacked in God's will and purpose. No one will disagree with me there. A spirit, when it is attacked, will do what is natural and primal. It will retaliate by faith!

*Romans 8:10: "... the Spirit is life because of righteousness."*

Your spirit desires to enforce the Grace of God! The spirit knoweth all things and, above all else, it knows that it has His Grace! The regenerated new creature in Christ would rather die than bow to evil! To the spirit person, to bow to evil is worse than death. It would be bowing to the spirit of death, the law of sin and death itself, sin consciousness!

In the spirit world where all things are conceived, it would be yielding its redemption to the law—undoing its own righteousness! The spirit is life because of righteousness, and it will not submit without the good fight of faith! The spirit person knows that the good fight of faith is its victory. To acquiesce unrighteously is to surrender to evil! To the spirit, that is total oppression. That is surrendering to darkness.

Your resurrected spirit of God is here to fight the good fight! Your spirit person (who you are in Christ) has special predestined battles it is prepared to take, different missions where these battles will be available. These battles are opportunities for advancement.

The spirit person does not want to hang around and "be nice." It wants to connect deeply with God and other like-minded folks

and have total victory over deceptions that are blocking its way
—joyfully and in warrior-like stance, picking up its cross and following its master's footsteps, being like Jesus, the image and
likeness of God, rebuking and rebutting evil.

## Without Vision, My People Perish

The true definition of depression is being out of spiritual purpose, taking a small piece of the pie. Staying alive is insufficient;
take what God has given you! Don't settle for less. Settling is
compromise, and your spirit would never indulge such victimization.

You are here for a divine and expansive purpose, one of
which is to live life very large. The larger you can live, the less
opportunity the old nature has to trap and deceive you. Living
large is a weapon in the spirit. It is a demonstration of your confidence in God's love and grace. When you are feeling insignifi-
cant in the bigger picture, less than divinely competent, you
have the option to retaliate! Step out, pick up your sword,
beloved, and strike, and you will be joyful beyond your wildest
dreams. You will be supernaturally upheld.

> *Ephesians 3:11: "According to the eternal purpose*
> *which he purposed in Christ Jesus our Lord."*

## How the Law Sees It (Sin Consciousness)

The Spirit of Condemnation wants you to identify the problem as your mistake; as if you are a guilty and condemned sinner. It is blaming you, talking to you as if you are the carnal old
creature! You are not this generational seed! As far as the east is
from the west is this seed nigh thee.

> *Psalm 103:12: "As far as the east is from the west,*
> *so far hath he removed our transgressions from us."*

## Receiving Grace

You receive your grace by faith, and that faith is your entrance into the Kingdom of God. By this grace, you are made the righteousness of God in Christ, the new creature in Christ, redeemed from the wiles of the law!

You want to stay in your position of power, demonstrating your grace by faith — retaliation faith, the faith that knows who you are, knows what He did for you, and knows your authority on this Earth in Jesus' name. Count it all joy when you get attacked, because you are about to gain. Not by suffering, not by hanging around praying for a miracle. No, by being you. You know what to do. You are the spirit person of a living God. When you get attacked, kick a little butt. *Don't just stand and try to get back what's been taken; you are being duped into wasting your time! Move on and take more. Tax the devil whenever you can!*

*Tax … Tax … Tax …*

## The Prize of the High Calling of God (Philippians 3:13-14)

God says press on, take what was taken and then add some interest. Take more. *Make the opposition suffer for attacking you, and stop these unrighteous attacks!*

*God is not teaching you through attacks;* God has given you His grace and His sword to enforce your authority and dominion! You will grow with God in the battlefield. Your spirit and heart will enlarge and your flesh decrease as you mortify these erroneous deeds of the impostor. *You will train the old creature to think twice before it dumps some disease or leads you to a wrong plan, some beguiling misadventure.* Stay awake in the game of life, and don't allow the old nature and its generational deceptions to take you out!

## Take What's Yours

The price has been paid for your grace, your dominion. You do not have to do anything to get it; just know that you have it and enforce His grace. Start an "Enforcing His Grace" group in your home. You will be amazed at the miracles that will happen when a few like-minded "Retaliators" get together!

There is absolutely nothing wrong with you! You are the new, improved you! God has fixed you entirely, from head to toe. You have been redone, changed, made new, better, complete! Leave yourself alone. Learn to recognize "self-fixing" as a hint, an omen, to take authority.

## Grace Tune-Up

When the enemy of your true identity wants to fix you, take a grace tune-up, and move on … As you start spending more time in the dispensation of grace, all the qualities you wanted to expand will be demonstrating themselves through you in your life.

*You already have it. You are already there. Don't settle for small fruit.*

> *Matthew 13:12: "For whosoever hath, to him shall be given, and he shall have more abundance: but whosoever hath not, from him shall be taken away even that he hath."*

# Chapter 40

## My Last Idol Revealed: Idols of the Impostor (Works)

The impostor will do anything to distract you from faith and purpose, distract you from moving ahead. The more advanced you get, the sneakier the counterfeit will be. Your opponent knows the importance of the "appointed time" and will watch and wait to deceive you. The impostor knows that you are learning how to take authority over it, that you have God-given power to do so. It has its position; it knows its job detail very well! It has to keep you ignorant of your dominion! The impostor has to keep you stuck, jammed, ignorant of its devices at all times! It knows that, if you are not moving on, you can be lost or tossed into an old way. It hopes that it can deceive you into being moved back and oppressing your faith. It thrives on your holding on to the past.

The impostor loves to keep you in an old spiritual purpose, yesterday's manna. It knows that only when you are led by God to your new day, your new manna, your sacred new moment, are you kept safe from its sabotage and wiles!

## The Impostor Wants You Out of Grace (The Power of God)

One of the deceptive ways the impostor has successfully used for centuries is to keep humans immobilized, to keep you in a repetitive position. You, the righteousness of God, can be diminished by deception to be nothing more than a parrot if you do not stay awake.

The impostor would like to keep you looking back, or staying stuck. Looking back is chasing doubt and agreeing with condemnation! Staying jammed is not letting go, nor is obsessing over a problem, trying to move ahead by plotting and planning, but actually not moving at all!

The impostor knows you cannot move ahead in your mind; you cannot work it out. There is no faith in it! No faith, no grace. A step must be taken. A step of faith is the solution! The awakened regenerated spirit is a warrior trained by God Himself to be aware of the wiles of evil. The regenerated spirit is a cool slayer of evil. It is not an intellectual reader of the one hundred ways to get to God. It scoffs at such attempts to undermine its authority!

The regenerated spirit is full in God and has the fullness of the Kingdom of God. It doesn't have to get anywhere or do anything to get what God has already fully given it. That is just another deception! Your spirit will not be conned by erroneous identification. The regenerated spirit is a Ghostbuster at its finest!

## Impostor Warfare

I will share a story of my own impostor deceiving me into six months of disobedience to God, six months of being tossed and confused. Six months of unconsciousness, of being deceived by the sneakiness of the counterfeit into idol worship.

## Holy Spirit Development

*Titus 3:5: "… by the washing of regeneration and renewing of the Holy Ghost."*

There was a time in my life when God was teaching me my ministry; it was a joyous time. I was very excited to be filled with the Holy Spirit, to be able to pray myself up into the spirit and enter into the Kingdom of God.

I was learning how to pray, cast out evil and always have spirit power, and stay above the flesh. I was getting authority over the old creature.

I wanted more and more of God: His intimacy, His power. As most sincere believers do, I wanted to please Him. I spent hours a day praying, reading the word, confessing scripture, and casting out principalities (deceptions) from myself. I was grounding in God and developing my ministry.

It was a blissful time of separation and sanctification! Most of my time was spent gloriously enjoying the Lord and learning His ways. I was high in the Lord, and was learning how to walk in the spirit. I was having deliverance meetings in my home in the evenings, and many people were being healed and delivered! We were all experiencing miracles and having a grand time growing in the Lord! The Lord was meeting us every step of the way ... We were exactly where we were supposed to be, led by God, enjoying our spiritual fruits!

## A Season of Spiritual Insurance

This went on for a season — about two years. I loved this time: I would prepare for a meeting, casting out generational deceptions in myself. I would keep casting till I sat in Heavenly places in Christ Jesus. I had no bad days. I was being sanctified via deliverance!

I was confident — never to be oppressed again. I had "up" insurance, Resurrection Blue Cross, Calvary Cross insurance. If anything got in my way, I cast it out! No matter what happened, how awful my day was, if any alleged transferring spirits remained from the meeting the night before, I cast them out! My days were spent identifying evil, praying, praising the Lord and in His Word.

I was living way above my natural condition and experienced no depression, no pain, no negative thoughts, no anger or fears. Anything daring to cling to my free spirit would simply be

281

cast out. I was getting a lot of deliverance practice — I was my own best customer! As soon as I would identify and cast a deception out, I would be separate from it — I could see what it really was, have a laugh, and return to my joy in the Lord.

*Ephesians 1:3: "Blessed be God the father of our Lord Jesus Christ, who hath blessed us with all spiritual blessings in heavenly places in Christ."*

## A Cast Machine

I became an energetic cast machine. I had deliverance mania. I got good at it. I could identify a spirit and separate it by its very thoughts! I could cast out one spirit, a ruling prince, and take hundreds of deceptions with it. I could cast out schizophrenia (double mindedness) with the Word of God! People were being healed of severe mental disorders by the power of God!

I had the power of the Holy Ghost to cast out diseases! I had the knowledge of His blood, His name, and had gained in my consecration, His anointing. I had seen so many principalities in all the self-casting I had done, that these deceptions were bowing to me rapidly! I had learned so much, directly from God himself. The Lord had taught me deliverance at another level of understanding. I was able to identify and cast out unwanted thoughts and behaviors, to take them right out of the mind.

The power of God has been underestimated in the deliverance ministry. Jesus is an incredible psychiatrist. All I had to do was know that it was all a lie ... I was soon able to cast unwanted perceptions out corporately and deliver the entire church with one simple cast. *The Lord Jesus Christ has given us power to cast out even the errors and deceptions in our carnal minds!* This sure beat being a therapist! To think that I used to sit there all day and listen to the impostor disclose all its problems.

## Why End This?

This was a special time; I didn't want it to end. Why would it end — this was as good as it gets! This was as high as any human being could desire to be. If I could bottle this, I could cure the world of cocaine addiction and end all oppressions. I had so much joy. I had arrived. I was living and being the spirit woman, separated from my past. By a few good casts a day, I could keep evil away ...

> *Ephesians 3:10: "To the intent now unto the principalities and powers in heavenly places might be known by the church the manifold wisdom of God."*

## Don't Get Good at It

I have noticed one very consistent thing with God — everything changes, everything ends, everything transmutes ... transforms. Once you have mastered "your way," it's time to move on! There will be the next thing to master, to learn, and to grow in grace.

> *Ecclesiastes 3:11: "He hath made every thing beautiful in His time: also he hath set the world in their heart, so that no man can find out the work that God maketh from the beginning to the end."*

## What God Wants

One thing that the Lord wants above all else is for us to grow in grace. We are ultimately on a grace journey. We will be asked to let go of everything till we walk just by faith. Grace is by faith! Faith in what? Faith in letting go of everything and being able to walk into the new moment of God, knowing that he will give you what you need. To be led by the spirit and new moment of God is the same thing. The trick is that the new moment can only be gotten by faith. There are carrots along the

way, but, ultimately, the new moment is by faith. No agenda —
no one hundred to do's — no right way, no wrong way.

God's way is simply the new moment by faith. That's where
the real miracles are. To walk by faith, one must take authority
over the old nature. Walking by faith and choosing to retaliate is
entering into the fire of sanctification with Jesus. It is a way to
gain authority over the old nature. Perhaps the only way.

## Faith in the New Moment

Faith in the new moment is very refined faith; it is faith that
believes God will provide for you, wherever you are, exactly
what you need. It is the laying down of your own understanding. All you have to do is lay it down. Take no thought and then
do not pick it up! It is the surrender of your mind unto the Lord.
Surrendering to God is the surrender of your mind — a bringing
of every thought into captivity to the obedience of Christ. (2
Corinthians 10:5) You cannot surrender "your life" without first
surrendering your mind, your thoughts. Your thought life.
Thought by thought ...

> 1 Corinthians 1:19: "For it is written, I will
> destroy the wisdom of the wise, and will bring
> to nothing the understanding of the prudent."

Faith in the new moment is your ability to walk into any situation and know that God is in it! To trust in God for everything!
Your old nature is the direct opposite of you. The carnal intellect
desires to work everything out, bringing everything eventually to
works, producing an intellectual idol. It is all a plot.

Idols of the mind (thoughts) plotting and scheming to do
"something" to get there, pondering and worrying without taking
the step towards the new direction, is a clever unidentified
deception of evil to hold you back. It's a premeditated mind
control jam. This is often diagnosed as anxiety. Don't fall for it.
You have power over it! When you are in one of the mind con-

trol jams, a mental conflict, or even indecision (a "should I or shouldn't I") take an action of faith. God will direct you! Faith pleases God. Faith evokes God!

> *Hebrews 11:6: "Without faith it is impossible to please Him."*

> *Galatians 5:4: "Christ is become of no effect unto you, whosoever of you are justified by the law; ye are fallen from grace."*

## My Stage of Glory

What the Lord wanted to accomplish at this time was to eliminate all of my works. Get me out of my house, out of my head, out of my studies and into the action of life. Not the works of sanctification, but the trials and tribulations of life would sanctify me via faith! This would be the arena where I would grow. Life itself was to be my stage of glory!

> *James 1:12: "Blessed is the man that endureth temptation: for when he is tried, he shall receive the crown of life, which the Lord hath promised to them that love Him."*

## A Step toward Purpose

To walk by faith is to just move ahead, without the impostor's mind directing you — just a walking towards purpose, positioning yourself to take any step towards purpose. "He who hath promised will bring your purpose to pass." This, my brothers and sisters, is the shortcut.

> *Galatians 2:21: "I do not frustrate the grace of God: for if righteousness come by the law, then Christ is dead in vain."*

## A Stumbling Block

I was so gung ho, so enthusiastic, and so sincere in my desire to work my way to heaven, to get more of God, that I

285

could not see that the season had changed! I was, however, starting to get some strong indications that I was moving in a wrong direction.

> Romans 9:32: *"Wherefore? because they sought it not by faith, but as it were by the works of the law. For they stumbled at that stumbling stone."*

## Losing My Insurance

There are two basic reasons for an attack, for a continuous oppression: you are either in God's perfect will and being opposed, held back from a great purpose, or you are out of purpose completely. I was losing my high. I would do my casting, praying, praising, but without the same results.

Sometimes I would go up in the spirit, feel elevated, but my insurance was no longer consistent. I had bad days — days when I would cast and cast and end up nauseous or oppressed! I considered the fact that I might be in works, but the impostor made a very strong argument. Perhaps you have heard this one yourself.

## The Debate
## (Words of Temptation)

"How can you be in works? You are in the Holy Spirit. God would not anoint this if it were not His purpose. You could not get an anointing out of God's will!"

That made perfect sense to me. Of course one could not. God only anoints His purpose. What is wrong with this picture? I was once high from casting out my own negative and generationally unwanted thoughts and replacing these thoughts with the Word of God ... Now it seemed as if every time I did something of God besides minister to others, I would have less of God.

## A New Way

Could God be asking me to do something else to keep myself separate from the flesh? What could be higher than this? I spent a lot of time learning the ways of the spirit. It was my ministry. I was a deliverance minister. A deliverance minister who could not cast something out of herself ... strange.

The whole thing was beyond my comprehension. There was no other way to separate myself if I were attacked, oppressed or deceived, so I continued. Things continued to worsen. Something was not right. I was feeling it strongly. I was out of the flow.

## There Is, Therefore, Now

The interesting thing about being out of purpose is that the attack I was getting from being out of purpose was more out of purpose than whatever purpose I was out of. If I miss a mark, God does not punish me. God would instruct me, correct me gently; whereas the out of purpose attack is the spirit of condemnation, another impostor deception. The impostor was simultaneously deceiving me into continuing to do something that was over, and attacking me with the spirit of condemnation for doing it.

*Romans 7:24: "O wretched man that I am!
Who shall deliver me from the body of this death?"*

*Romans 8:1: "There is therefore now no
condemnation to them which are in Christ Jesus,
who walk not after the flesh, but after the Spirit."*

## When in Doubt, Play It Out

*James 1:8: "A double minded man is unstable in all his ways."*

The attack began creating conflict in my mind. Was it condemnation? Was it God? Should I continue? Should I give it up?

287

You know the routine. I had to know, one way or the other. I had to be sure, to find out where God truly was in this whole scenario, and I had to stop the attack. I made a decision … I would take action. I would up the ante! We have a saying in my ministry: "When in doubt, play it out." I chose to play it out!

## Holy Ghost Marathon

I constructed a plan. I would take a long weekend, do all my works — shoot my entire works arsenal. I would fast for four days, pray, worship, confess scripture, and cast out error. I would do a four-day works marathon. At the end of four days, I would know! I would have either broken through the attack if it was one and feel great, my joy restored, or I would not break through and I would be certain that this season in my life was over…

## My Plan in Action

I began as usual, in the middle of my living room, the same room in which I held the deliverance meetings.

I would first walk around the huge space (which had minimal furniture for ministry purposes) and just pray in the spirit. Then I would put my praise music on, as I did this day. I praised and prayed in the spirit till I felt the anointing of the Holy Spirit. I then began my usual manner of calling out and casting unwanted spirits out. Once I was separated by the praise and praying, I could easily perceive where error was attempting to distract me and where spirit was leading!

## Spiritual Works???

That's what made this situation so difficult to discern. It seemed that, even if I were out of the Lord's leading, out of my personal purpose, the spirit still had authority over the flesh and the battle still had the power of God!

*Mark 1:27: "For with authority commandeth he*
*even the unclean spirits, and they do obey him."*

I started getting some hints by the second day which way this was going, but I had to go all the way. I had to be sure. I was getting concerned.

How would I keep myself above my flesh without my process? How would I stay in the spirit? The impostor was using a "wondering" interrogation as its defensive posture. The inquiring flesh wanted to know. Evil wanted to jam my mind.

Three days and nights unfolded and I still had not broken through, but one never knows in a spiritual battle. Just when you think it's over, things can change. I had to see it through till I was sure — till there was not one unanswered question, till I knew one way or another … till I was single-minded.

*Matthew 6:22: "If therefore thine eye be*
*single, thy whole body shall be full of light."*

## The Fourth Day

I was not in the spirit anymore. The more works I did, the lower I got. By the fourth day, I was sick, literally shaking and sick. It was clear that I was moving in a wrong direction. I had my answer.

*Romans 4:4: "Now to him that worketh is the*
*reward not reckoned of grace, but of debt."*

## How Long, Lord?

The question changed. I was no longer asking if I were moving in a wrong direction. That was clear. It was how long. How long had I been off my path? How long had I been deceived? How long had I been out of God's will and purpose?

I was heartsick, disgusted. How could this be? The impostor chimed in to kick me when I was down, and I was literally down. I was lying down flat on my living room floor, unable to get up, weakened, oppressed and very shaken.

What did I have to call my own? Everything I believed in had just fallen apart — all of my religion, my good works, down the drain. I was a person out of God's will, on my own agenda. I had no truth. The impostor took this opportune moment to finish me off entirely. "You have no truth," the impostor declared. "You have nothing left to believe in!"

My heart cried out to God, "Lord, this was about you. Truly, this was about you!"

I had lost my concern for how I would be upheld in the spirit without works. I had a change of heart! I was heartbroken; I had betrayed my Love. All that was important to me now was to clarify my intent with the lover of my soul.

"Lord," I cried, "I wanted to get closer to you. I have gotten further away. What I wanted was more of you. This was all about you, Lord."

The impostor took another shot. "You are so depressed," it commented. "You have no truth!"

"Shut up!" I said. There was no point in my going there now. "That's a downhill road, and I am not going there! No, not now. I am not that deceived." I quickly identified that line of thought and knew that this was no time to fellowship with more evil ... no point in receiving more victimization now ... I needed God. I could not afford the luxury of listening to the impostor now. I had listened long enough. "Just shut up," I said again. "No more!

My heart was stronger in its concern over the loss of my connection to its love. The threats of the flesh, the confusion, nothing mattered anymore but Jesus ... my Jesus.

## "I" Began to Think

I began to think in my spirit mind. "What truth do I have? What still stands? What do I know? What is true for me, even now at this low point? Do I have one thing in my heart of hearts, one totally authentic reality? Is it all a sham, a total deception?

"One truth. I need one truth. What do I really know? What cannot be taken away from me? One word. What do I have absolute faith in?

"Do I have one truth that my heart agrees with? Not mental ascent, not works? What do I know that I know to be fact?"

## I Know One Thing ...

As I searched my heart for this assurance, I felt myself start to rise. I was getting up off the floor. My spirit was being stirred. I felt a surge of power. I was standing now, hearing my own words come out of my mouth. These words were not oppressed; they were full of faith. They came from a very deep place in my spirit.

They answered my question. "I know one thing," my spirit declared. "Whatever happened here today, whatever has been going on, no matter how far off I have been, no matter how long ..." I started standing a little taller, my eyes on Jesus, and my spirit continued. "I know one thing ..."

Yes, I had a truth. "My sins are forgiven, and your grace is sufficient."

In a second, I was totally delivered, in great joy, not at all sick or oppressed. My truth had broken me through.

I said it again gratefully, joyfully, crying in the glory of it. Yes, it was a fact. "My sins are forgiven, and your grace is sufficient!"

The only thing in my body that had not been healed up to that point was a neck inflammation, a chronic condition. On x-rays, it was diagnosed as an arthritic neck. I had this pain for over twenty years. Even as a child, I had had a special pillow, and still used a tiny little foam pillow to sleep on. I needed to be very careful how I positioned my neck, no turning to the left, etc. To be honest, I almost always had neck pain. I had prayed, cast, gotten prayer, etc. ... I still had neck pain.

This time, as I spoke my one solitary truth, repeating it gleefully, "Your grace is sufficient, my sins are forgiven!" I felt something fly out of my neck. Yes, "a something" flew out! My neck was healed, my neck was free ... The only thing that had the power to deliver my neck was His absolute grace, and my total acceptance of it.

*2 Corinthians 12:9: "And he said to me, My grace is sufficient for thee: for my strength is made perfect in weakness."*

## I Said His Grace Is Sufficient

In the following days, when this neck pain would attempt to return, I would go in front of a big mirror, look at my neck and repeat myself, saying factually, simply, calmly, no yelling, no screaming, no praying, no casting, just speaking the truth again, "His grace is sufficient," and it would leave again ... It has never returned.

I have found grace to be the hardest lesson, the most difficult thing to receive, the free gift of grace that has within itself the fullness of the power of God.

*To enforce this amazing grace, all we have to know is that our sins are forgiven and His grace is sufficient. (2 Corinthians 12:9)*

## A Retaliator Is a Grace Enforcer, Armed and Dangerous!

*John 1:16-17: "And of his fullness have all we received, grace for grace. For the law was given by Moses, but grace and truth came by Jesus Christ."*

For this, I give Him praise!

## *The End*

CPSIA information can be obtained
at www.ICGtesting.com
Printed in the USA
FSOW03n0458301117
41522FS